611291

Protecting
Huma
Subjec

Protecting Human Subjects

Departmental Subject Pools and Institutional Review Boards

Edited by
GARVIN CHASTAIN AND
R. ERIC LANDRUM

American Psychological Association
Washington, DC

First Printing March 1999

Second Printing April 2002
Published by
American Psychological Association
750 First Street, NE
Washington, DC 20002

Copies may be ordered from
APA Order Department
P.O. Box 92984
Washington, DC 20090-2984

In the UK and Europe, copies may be ordered from
American Psychological Association
3 Henrietta Street
Covent Garden, London
WC2E 8LU England

Typeset in Palatino by EPS Group Inc., Easton, MD

Printer: Edwards Brothers, Ann Arbor, MI
Cover Designer: Kaelin Chappell, San Diego, CA
Editor/Project Manager: Debbie K. Hardin, Reston, VA

Library of Congress Cataloging-in-Publication Data
Protecting human subjects : departmental subject pools and institutional
    review boards / edited by Garvin Chastain and R. Eric Landrum.
        p.   cm.
    Includes bibliographical references and index.
    ISBN 1-55798-575-8
    1. Human experimentation in psychology—Moral and ethical
aspects.   2. Psychology—Research—Moral and ethical aspects.
I. Chastain, Garvin D.   II. Landrum, R. Eric.
BF181.P65   1999
174′.915—dc21   99-22348
                                                                          CIP

British Library Cataloguing-in-Publication Data
A CIP record is available from the British Library

Printed in the United States of America

Contents

Contributors

Laura L. Bowman, *Department of Psychology, Central Connecticut State University*

Darrell L. Butler, *Department of Psychological Sciences, Ball State University*

Garvin Chastain, *Department of Psychology, Boise State University*

James R. Council, *Department of Psychology, North Dakota State University*

Janet F. Gillespie, *Department of Psychology, SUNY College at Brockport*

Brian A. Gladue, *Department of Psychology, University of Cincinnati*

Jessica Kaster-Bundgaard, *Department of Psychology, North Dakota State University*

R. Eric Landrum, *Department of Psychology, Boise State University*

Richard L. Moreland, *Department of Psychology, University of Pittsburgh*

Gregory L. Murphy, *Department of Psychology, University of Illinois*

Joan E. Sieber, *Department of Psychology, California State University-Hayward*

Elizabeth J. H. Smith, *Department of Psychology, North Dakota State University*

Bradley M. Waite, *Department of Psychology, Central Connecticut State University*

Michael W. Wiederman, *Department of Psychological Sciences, Ball State University*

Preface

This volume offers information to researchers and scholars about the appropriate treatment of human subjects[1] in psychological research. The chapter authors deal with the issues and concerns of researchers and those interested in research regarding how human subjects are protected, emphasizing the roles of departmental subject pools and institutional review boards in this process. We address practical issues in conducting research with human subjects as well as in protecting members of unique subject populations. This volume will be useful for those currently conducting research as well as for those planning to implement a research program. Each chapter provides an empirically based treatment of issues ranging from data collection details to institution-wide concerns.

Departmental subject pools (DSPs) provide an opportunity for university researchers to explore experimental hypotheses by testing groups of human participants selected in a relatively organized, efficient way. Typically, students enrolled in undergraduate courses are given the opportunity to experience experimental research firsthand through their participation as members of the department's human subject pool. Researchers bear the responsibility of weighing the costs and benefits of participation to ensure the protection of each subject. This volume outlines relevant considerations in these respects and offers new approaches on how to improve interactions among institutions, departments, researchers, and participants.

Institutional Review Boards (IRBs) also are responsible for the protection of human subjects. A university IRB is a group

---

Throughout this book we refer to human *subjects,* as opposed to *research participants.* The American Psychological Association recommends the use of the latter term to avoid objectifying those involved in research. However, we have used *subjects* because this continues to be common terminology among institutions and thus serves as a term of art in context.

of individuals, usually some from the academic community and others from off campus, who evaluate projects proposed by researchers and decide for each project whether it meets certain standards regarding the ethical treatment of human participants. Although the IRB oversight function is vital to the process, IRBs may seem to have concerns that differ from those of researchers. This volume addresses many of those concerns and offers suggestions on how researchers and IRBs can work together more effectively in pursuing their joint goal of advancing science and protecting human subjects.

The impetus for this volume was a symposium that was held at the Midwestern Psychological Association meeting in Chicago, Illinois, in May of 1995. Following the symposium there was general agreement about the need for an edited volume directed at surveying current practices and trends regarding departmental subject pools and institutional review boards at academic institutions. In addition, messages frequently posted to Internet bulletin boards, such as TIPS (Teaching in the Psychological Sciences), indicate that many who are interested in conducting research with human subjects now work at primarily undergraduate institutions where no human subject pool has ever existed. In this way, then, this project fills a void in the literature. We have chosen topics that are reflective of the diversity of current subject pool and institutional review board policies and practices, and thus are relevant to a variety of people with related interests.

It is our intention that the resources provided by this volume should be used by anyone who interacts with or is concerned about the research process. More scholarly attention needs to be turned to the ethics and efficiency of our practices. If we are able to stimulate greater interest and attention to the treatment of human participants in psychological research, then we will have met our goal.

Protecting
Human
Subjects

Introduction

R. Eric Landrum

Although variations exist, psychology is typically defined as the science of human behavior and thought processes (e.g., Lefton, 1997). Psychology as a "science" differs from other approaches of studying human behavior (e.g., philosophy) in its reliance on systematic methods of studying and measuring behavior, as well as in its dependence on empirical observations. Since the days of Wundtian psychology and structuralism, psychologists have been interested in the empirical observation of behavior through the use of systematic research methods. In those early days, the technique was primarily introspection, and the subjects (now called *participants*) were the researchers themselves, examining the structural components of their own minds. As structuralism faded away, to be replaced by functionalism and behaviorism, the emphasis shifted from the observation of internal behavior (i.e., introspection) to the observation of external, directly observable behaviors. This shift focused attention on the behavior of others. Thus other people and sometimes animals became the "subjects" of study. This systematic study of others has survived behaviorism, neobehaviorism, and the cognitive revolution. In the current study of human subjects (participants), other people play a key role in attempting to understand human behavior and thought processes.

Psychologists have a unique and perhaps paradoxical role in this endeavor. Our goal is to better understand human behavior and to develop ways through which we might improve the human condition. However, we "study" and "experiment" on these same human participants to understand basic human functions as well as develop intervention-type approaches (e.g., therapeutic approaches). We study those individuals whom we ultimately wish to help, wish to educate, and wish to enlighten. It would seem, at least implicitly, that

3

we have an ethical obligation to protect those whom we study. Surprisingly, very little was mentioned in the literature about protecting human subjects until the aftermath of World War II (Office for Protection From Research Risks [OPRR], 1993), although occasionally the protection of human subjects was referred to (Wieman, 1922).

Following the discovery of the Nazi atrocities committed during World War II, the Nuremberg Military Tribunal issued a list of 10 guidelines for the involvement of human beings in research; these guidelines are today called the Nuremberg Code (Trials of War Criminals Before the Nuremberg Military Tribunals Under Control Council Law No. 10, 1949). The Nuremberg Code established such standards as voluntary and informed consent, freedom from coercion, scientific value of research, and the right to withdraw from research at any time. World War II, its aftermath, and subsequent documents did stimulate a discussion in psychology about research ethics and the protection of human subjects (Berg, 1954; Shimkin, Guttentag, Kidd, & Johnson, 1953), and the Nuremberg Code today continues to influence experimentation (Alexander, 1976; Freedman, 1987; Stuart, 1978; Young, 1998). The American Psychological Association (APA) developed its own code of research ethics in 1953, and it is periodically updated.

Other formal recommendations followed the Nuremberg Code. In 1964 the 18th World Medical Assembly in Helsinki, Finland, adopted the Declaration of Helsinki: Recommendations Guiding Medical Doctors in Biomedical Research Involving Human Subjects (OPRR, 1993). As did the Nuremberg Code, the Declaration of Helsinki stimulated more efforts to understand the impact of experimentation involving humans (Allenbeck, 1997; Burke, 1985; Gutteridge, Bankowski, Curran, & Dunne, 1982).

In the United States, the regulations to protect human subjects were introduced in May 1974 and disseminated by the Department of Health, Education and Welfare. This formalized and raised to regulatory status the National Institute of Health's Policies for the Protection of Human Subjects, which were issued in 1966 (OPRR, 1993). In July 1974 the National

Research Act established a commission to identify the basic ethical guidelines that should be used in research and to develop a method to ensure their use. This commission issued a report defining these basic ethical principles and a mechanism for their enforcement in what is known as the Belmont Report (National Commission for the Protection of Human Subjects in Biomedical and Behavioral Research, 1979). These regulations established the Institutional Review Board (IRB) as one mechanism to protect human subjects. The recommendations of the Belmont Report are formally listed in Title 45, Part 46, of the Code of Federal Regulations (referred to in legal notation as 45 C.F.R. 46). The Belmont Report and IRB regulations continue to be influential in the conduct of research in the United States. This book examines those critical issues and processes related to the protection of human subjects who participate in research.

We approach this topic with an interest in the empirical research that has been done to study the effects of the practice of research. From the standpoint of metacognition, this is a volume about the research done on the effects of conducting research. The two primary mechanisms that govern the processes of conducting human subjects research are the departmental subject pool on the local level and the Institutional Review Board on the institutional level. The goal of this volume is to examine these issues from a number of relevant perspectives. Prior to previewing the specific chapters of this volume, a review of the research on department subject pools and IRBs is in order. After a review of the literature, two clear trends emerge: (a) the IRB process has been studied much more frequently than the subject pool process, and (b) neither area has had much empirical research conducted concerning its operations. This book aims to fill that void.

Department Subject Pools (DSPs)

Given the history of empirical research in psychology (preceding the introduction of IRBs in the 1970s by decades), one might expect a rich literature that addresses the recruitment and protection of human subjects who participate in psychological research. But that is not the case. The literature that does exist can be divided into three areas: (a) national surveys on subject pool practices and recruitment, (b) regulations and management of subject pools, and (c) general issues related to obtaining subjects.

National surveys of psychology departments have been conducted by Miller (1981) and Sieber and Saks (1989) in the United States, by Lindsay and Holden (1987) in Canada, and by Diamond and Reidpath (1992) in Australia. (Miller's work also included some universities from Canada and the United Kingdom.) These studies help us to understand the normative processes of subject pool operation, and comparatively, help to delineate subject pool practices that may be more culture-specific. Additional work has been conducted in the area of DSP regulations and management by de Sola Pool (1983) and McCord (1991). Johnson (1973) and Smith and Leigh (1997) have written about the issues and challenges in recruiting subjects. (Smith & Leigh, 1997, deal with how new technology such as the Internet influences the recruitment of subjects across new media.) Taken together, however, this literature is surprisingly limited for an enterprise (i.e., the subject pool) that generates so much research productivity annually.

We seek to address the functioning of subject pools directly. In chapter 1, Landrum and Chastain report on a national study of undergraduate-only departments of psychology, revealing some of the current practices and procedures used around the country. They also report on some of the more innovative approaches some universities are using to ensure a learning experience for research participants. In chapter 2, one of the best-known scholars in the field of studying and understanding ethics and IRB functioning, Joan Sieber, looks at the practices that make a subject pool ethical or unethical. She points out "best practices" that subject pool administrators should be aware of and provides advice for those wishing to ensure ethical subject pool practices.

Institutional Review Boards (IRBs)

When examining the literature on IRBs, the sheer volume of research on this topic is impressive. Although space constraints prevent a thorough discussion of all the related literature, we will attempt to provide a comprehensive review of the areas of IRB scholarship and appropriate references to that literature. For organizational purposes, the IRB literature is divided into sections. These sections are (a) the IRB and specific research populations; (b) the IRB and specific research topics; (c) day-to-day functioning of the IRB; (d) the use of ethical guidelines and the protection from harm by the IRB; (e) informed consent issues and confidentiality; and (f) miscellaneous and general issues for IRBs to consider, including practices and procedures. A review of each of these areas follows, accompanied by references to the relevant literature. Sieber (1992) has provided a good overview for IRBs in the planning and conduct of ethically responsible research.

The IRB and Specific Research Populations

Part of the role of the IRB is to pay special attention to protecting those subject populations that may have difficulty protecting themselves (Fisher, 1997; Fletcher, Dommel, & Cowell, 1985). This need for additional attention may be because of some sort of behavioral anomaly (e.g., Alzheimer's disease) or some sort of behavioral situation or consequence (e.g., a prisoner in a corrections facility). Although the IRB has a wide-ranging group of individuals to protect, the literature mentions groups such as children and adolescents (Ackerman, 1995; Amiel, 1985; Leikin, 1993; Mammel & Kaplan, 1995; Phillips, 1994; Porter, 1995; Rogers, D'Angelo, & Futterman, 1994; Scott-Jones, 1994; Sieber, 1994a; Theut & Kohrman, 1990), African Americans (Harris, 1996), family studies (Parker & Lidz, 1994), prisoners in correctional facilities (Glueck, 1931; Megargee, 1995; Reilly, 1991), senior citizens (Long, 1982), Alzheimer's disease patients (High, 1993), medical students (Christakis, 1985), and psychiatric patients (DeRenzo, 1994; Miller & Rosenstein, 1997; Pinals, Malhotra,

Breier, & Pickar, 1998). Each of these subject populations has special needs and concerns to which IRBs must be sensitive.

We address some of these issues in the section Vulnerable Populations and Risk of Research. In chapter 8 James Council, Elizabeth Smith, Jessica Kaster-Bundgaard, and Brian Gladue investigate how IRBs view researchers who conduct research in areas with greater than minimal risk, as well as how researchers view the role and decision making of the IRB members. Other chapters, such as those by Joan Sieber (chapter 2) and Michael Wiederman (chapter 9) address issues related to working with protected populations in sensitive research areas.

The IRB and Specific Research Topics

It seems that certain areas of research also draw special attention from IRBs in their effort to protect human subjects. Most often mentioned in the literature are areas such as the study of hypnosis (Coe & Ryken, 1979; Council, Smith, Kaster-Bundgaard, & Gladue, 1997), clinical trials (Gordon, 1985; Meinert, 1998; Orr, 1996; Ortega & Dal-Re, 1995; Perry, 1987; Prentice et al., 1993; Shimm & Spece, 1992; Spilker, 1992), those with HIV or AIDS (Bayer, Levine, & Murray, 1984; Hammett & Dubler, 1990; Landesman, 1986; Leikin, 1989; Levine, Dubler, & Levine, 1991; Meyers & Dunton, 1988; Novick, 1984; Porter, Glass, & Koff, 1989), neurobiological (Shamoo, 1997), and even archival research (Taube & Burkhardt, 1997). These types of research areas often draw additional attention because of their potential sensitivity.

In chapter 9 Michael Wiederman examines one area of research not often mentioned in the IRB literature: sexuality research. Studying sensitive topics such as sexuality heightens the IRB's attention to issues such as informed consent, emotional trauma, confidentiality, and the right to withdraw from a study. In addition, researchers do not want to add to the discomfort of participants nor experience high nonresponse rates, yet these are real concerns in highly sensitive areas of research.

The Day-to-Day Functioning of IRBs

Although special populations and particular research topics draw added attention from IRBs, the board's charge is the protection of all human subjects (Edgar & Rothman, 1995; Schmidt & Meara, 1996; Sieber, 1989b). Some scholars have turned their attention to the day-to-day operations and procedures of how IRBs operate. Some of the research done in this area has examined how IRBs make judgments in the review of proposals (Ceci, Peters, & Plotkin, 1985; Chesapeake Research Review, 1995; Colombo, 1995; Freedman, 1987; Gordon & Prentice, 1997; Gray, Cooke, & Tannenbaum, 1978; Mordock, 1995; Pattullo, 1987; Reilly, 1991; Treadway & Rossi, 1977; Williams, 1984), the role of nonscientists or nonpsychologists as members of the IRB (Gilbert, 1985; Murray, 1984; Porter, 1986, 1987), and how the creation of federal policy influences IRB function (de Sola Pool, 1983; Grigsby & Roof, 1993; Porter, 1991).

The chapters by Gregory Murphy (chapter 6) and Janet Gillespie (chapter 7) address the issues of operations and procedures of IRBs in various types of institutional settings. Also, chapters by Darrell Butler (chapter 5), James Council and colleagues (chapter 8), and Michael Wiederman (chapter 9) address related issues.

The IRB, Ethical Guidelines, and Protecting Subjects From Harm

Ethical guidelines play a key role in how research functions (Green, Pascual-Leone, & Wasserman, 1997; Sieber, 1994b), and the IRB is a primary enforcement mechanism in protecting all human subjects from harm (Arnold et al. 1995; Fisher & Fyrberg, 1994; Lackey, 1986; Meslin, 1990; Reese & Fremouw, 1984; Rosenthal, 1995; Rosnow, Rotheram-Borus, Ceci, Blanck, & Koocher, 1993; Williams & Ouren, 1976). The explication of these roles has taken a number of forms in the literature, including how fraud and misconduct affect participants (Hilgartner, 1990), the research experiment from the participant's perspective (Dubler, 1986; Kalman, Talon,

Frances, & Kocsis, 1982; Landrum & Chastain, 1995; Prentice et al., 1993; Roberts, Newcomb, & Fost, 1993; Schreier & Stadler, 1992; White & Morse, 1988), and issues related to the conduct of research (Sieber, 1993), including the use of particular methodologies (Aguinis & Handelsman, 1997; Brickhouse, 1992; Cupples & Gochnauer, 1985; Marvin, 1985) and the payment of subjects (Ackerman, 1989; Macklin, 1989).

In chapter 3 Bradley Waite and Laura Bowman explore how participants feel in being a part of research, including the study of student attitudes, satisfaction, and attainment of knowledge. Richard Moreland's chapter 4 presents an organizational method of conducting research that systematically assesses and evaluates the learning experiences of students. In chapter 5 Darrell Butler addresses the problem of making sure that the participants show up to the study to participate, so both the researcher will benefit from the subject's participation and the subject can reap some of the educational benefits of participating in research. Other chapters of this volume also address practical matters in conducting research, including the chapters by Landrum and Chastain (chapter 1), Sieber (chapter 2), Murphy (chapter 6), and Gillespie (chapter 7).

Informed Consent and Confidentiality

A good deal of research effort in the study of IRBs has been devoted to the role of informed consent and confidentiality in research (Anderson, Jameton, Reitemeier, & Prentice, 1995; Angoff, 1984; Black & Hodge, 1987; Candilis, Wesley, & Wichman, 1993; Fletcher et al., 1985; Geller & Lidz, 1987; Mahler, 1986; Newton, 1984; Pinals et al., 1998; Powers, 1993; Reiser & Knudson, 1993; Silva & Sorrell, 1988; Taub, 1986; Tuthill, 1997). These two components of the research process can also be traced back to the development of the Nuremberg Code and the ultimate protection of human subjects. A newer area of research in this field involves not only the development of informed consent forms but also their readability and comprehension by research subjects (Hochauser, 1997; Lawson &

Adamson, 1995; Peterson, Clancy, Champion & McLarty, 1992; Waggoner & Mayo, 1995; Young, Hooker, & Freeberg, 1990).

In this volume both the chapters by Joan Sieber (chapter 2) and Michael Wiederman (chapter 9) address the issues of confidentiality and the ethical treatment of human subjects.

General Issues

There are many researchers who address general operational practices, such as the role the IRB plays in the sharing of scientific data (Sieber, 1989a) and the implications of the Belmont Report (Marshall, 1986).

The Scope of This Volume

This book has two objectives: (a) to present empirical data on the operations of department subject pools and institutional review boards; and (b) to expand the scholarship in the area of departmental subject pool structure and function.

This volume is designed to focus in on the key issues of the day in the protection of human subjects. We address practical issues, and we focus in on what departments in particular and universities in general need to know and do to administer a successful and ethical research program with human subjects.

References

Ackerman, T. F. (1989). An ethical framework for the practice of paying research subjects. *IRB: A Review of Human Subjects Research, 11*(4), 1–4.

Ackerman, T. F. (1995). The ethics of phase I pediatric oncology trials. *IRB: A Review of Human Subjects Research, 17*, 1–5.

Aguinis, H., & Handelsman, M. M. (1997). The unique ethical challenge of the bogus pipeline methodology: Let the data speak. *Journal of Applied Social Psychology, 27*, 582–587.

Alexander, L. (1976). Ethics of human experimentation. *Psychiatric Journal of the University of Ottawa, 1*, 40–46.

Allenbeck, P. (1997). Forensic psychiatric studies and research ethical considerations. *Nordic Journal of Psychiatry, 51*, 53–56, 73–95.

American Psychological Association. (1953). *Ethical standards of psychologists.* Washington, DC: Author.

Amiel, S. A. (1985). Pediatric research on diabetes: The problem of hospitalizing youthful subjects. *IRB: A Review of Human Subjects Research, 7*, 4–5.

Anderson, J. R., Jameton, A., Reitemeier, P. J., & Prentice, E. (1995). The case of two devices: Disclosure to subjects following Phase IV ("postmarketing") research. *IRB: A Review of Human Subjects Research, 17*, 6–9.

Angoff, N. R. (1984). An inadvertent breach of confidentiality. *IRB: A Review of Human Subjects Research, 6*, 5–6.

Arnold, L. E., Stoff, D. M., Cook, E., Cohen, D. J., Kruesi, M., Wright, C., Hattab, J., Graham, P., Zametkin, A., Castellanos, F. X., McMahan, W., & Leckman, J. F. (1995). Ethical issues in biological psychiatric research with children and adolescents. *Journal of the American Academy of Child and Adolescent Psychiatry, 34*, 929–939.

Bayer, R., Levine, C., & Murray, T. H. (1984). Guidelines for confidentiality in research on AIDS. *IRB: A Review of Human Subjects Research, 6*, 1–7.

Benson, P. R. (1989). The social control of human biomedical research: An overview and review of the literature. *Social Science & Medicine, 29*, 1–12.

Berg, I. A. (1954). The use of human subjects in psychological research. *American Psychologist, 9*, 108–111.

Black, K. J., & Hodge, M. H. (1987). Protecting subjects' identity in test–retest experiments. *IRB: A Review of Human Subjects Research, 9*, 10–11.

Brickhouse, N. W. (1992). Ethics in field–based research: Ethical principles and relational considerations. *Science Education, 76*, 93–103.

Burke, A. W. (1985). Mental health and apartheid: World Psychiatric Association conference report. *International Journal of Social Psychiatry, 31*, 144–148.

Candilis, P. J., Wesley, R. W., & Wichman, A. (1993). A survey of researchers using a consent policy for cognitively impaired human research subjects. *IRB: A Review of Human Subjects Research, 15*, 1–4.

Ceci, S. J., Peters, D., & Plotkin, J. (1985). Human subjects review, personal values, and the regulation of social science research. *American Psychologist, 40*, 994–1002.

Chesapeake Research Review. (1995). On being an IRB. *IRB: A Review of Human Subjects Research, 17*, 12–16.

Christakis, N. (1985). Do medical student research subjects need special attention? *IRB: A Review of Human Subjects Research, 7*, 1–4.

Coe, W. C., & Ryken, K. (1979). Hypnosis and risks to human subjects. *American Psychologist, 34*, 673–681.

Colombo, J. (1995). Cost, utility, and judgments of institutional review boards. *Psychological Science, 6*, 318–319.

Council, J. R., Smith, E. J. H., Kaster-Bundgaard, J., & Gladue, B. A. (1997). Ethical evaluation of hypnosis research: A survey of investigators and their Institutional Review Boards. *American Journal of Clinical Hypnosis, 39*, 258–265.

Cupples, B., & Gochnauer, M. (1985). The investigator's duty not to deceive. *IRB: A Review of Human Subjects Research, 7*, 1–6.

DeRenzo, E. G. (1994). The ethics in involving psychiatrically impaired persons in research. *IRB: A Review of Human Subjects Research, 16*, 7–9.

de Sola Pool, I. (1983). Human subjects regulations on the social sciences. *Annals of the New York Academy of Sciences, 403*, 101–110.

Diamond, M. R., & Reidpath, D. D. (1992). Psychology ethics down under: A survey of student subject pools in Australia. *Ethics & Behavior, 2*, 101–108.

Dubler, N. N. (1986). Treating research subjects fairly. *IRB: A Review of Human Subjects Research, 8*, 7–9.

Edgar, H., & Rothman, D. J. (1995). The institutional review board and beyond: Future challenges to the ethics of human experimentation. *Milbank Quarterly, 73*, 489–506.

Fisher, C. B. (1997). A relational perspective on ethics-in-science decision making for research with vulnerable populations. *IRB: A Review of Human Subjects Research, 19*, 1–4.

Fisher, C. B., & Fyrberg, D. (1994). Participant partners: College students weigh the costs and benefits of deceptive research. *American Psychologist, 49*, 417–427.

Fletcher, J. C., Dommel, F. W., & Cowell, D. D. (1985). Consent to research with impaired human subjects. *IRB: A Review of Human Subjects Research, 7*, 7–11.

Freedman, B. (1987). Scientific value and validity as ethical requirements for research: A proposed explication. *IRB: A Review of Human Subjects Research, 9*, 7–10.

Geller, J. L., & Lidz, C. W. (1987). When the subjects are hospital staff, is it ethical (or possible) to get informed consent? *IRB: A Review of Human Subjects Research, 9*, 4–5.

Gilbert, S. J. (1985). "The behavior of nonpsychologists on research review committee": Reply. *American Psychologist, 40*, 1265–1266.

Glueck, S. (1931). Mental hygiene and crime. *Psychoanalytic Review, 19*, 23–35.

Gordon, B., & Prentice, E. (1997). Continuing review of research involving human subjects: Approach to the problem and remaining areas of concern. *IRB: A Review of Human Subjects Research, 19*, 8–11.

Gordon, R. S. (1985). The design and conduct of randomized clinical trials. *IRB: A Review of Human Subjects Research, 7*, 12.

Gray, B. H., Cooke, R. A., & Tannenbaum, A. S. (1978). Research involving human subjects: The performance of institutional review boards is assessed in this empirical study. *Science, 201*, 1094–1101.

Green, R. M., Pascual-Leone, A., & Wasserman, E. M. (1997). Ethical guidelines for rTMS research. *IRB: A Review of Human Subjects Research, 19*, 1–7.

Grigsby, R. K., & Roof, H. L. (1993). Federal policy for the protection of human subjects: Application to research on social work practice. *Research on Social Work Practice, 3*, 448–461.

Gutteridge, F., Bankowski, Z., Curran, W., & Dunne, J. (1982). The structure and functioning of ethical review committees. *Social Science & Medicine, 16*, 1791–1800.

Hammett, T. M., & Dubler, N. N. (1990). Clinical and epidemiologic research on HIV infection and AIDS among correctional inmates: Regulation, ethics, and procedure. *Evaluation Review, 14*, 482–501.

Harris, J. L. (1996). Issues in recruiting African American participants for research. In A. G. Kamhi, K. E. Pollock, et al. (Eds.), *Communication development and disorders in African American children: Research, assessment, and intervention* (pp. 19–34). Baltimore: Brookes.

High, D. M. (1993). Advancing research with Alzheimer disease subjects: Investigators' perceptions and ethical issues. *Alzheimer Disease & Associated Disorders, 7*, 165–178.

Hilgartner, S. (1990). Research fraud, misconduct, and the IRB. *IRB: A Review of Human Subjects Research, 12*, 1–4.

Hochauser, M. (1997). Some overlooked aspects of consent form readability. *IRB: A Review of Human Subjects Research, 19*, 5–9.

Johnson, R. W. (1973). The obtaining of experimental subjects. *Canadian Psychologist, 14*, 208–211.

Kalman, T. P., Talon, N. S., Frances, A., & Kocsis, J. H. (1982). A controlled study of satisfaction among psychobiology research patients. *American Journal of Psychiatry, 139*, 344–347.

Lackey, D. P. (1986). A single subject in multiple protocols: Is the risk equitable? *IRB: A Review of Human Subjects Research, 8*, 8–10.

Landesman, S. H. (1986). The ethical obligations of research subjects to be informed of their HIV status. *IRB: A Review of Human Subjects Research, 8*, 9.

Landrum, R. E., & Chastain, G. (1995). Experiment spot-checks: A method for assessing the educational value of undergraduate participation in research. *IRB: A Review of Human Subjects Research, 17*, 4–6.

Lawson, S. L., & Adamson, H. M. (1995). Informed consent readability: Subject understanding of 15 common consent form phrases. *IRB: A Review of Human Subjects Research, 17*, 16–19.

Lefton, L. A. (1997). *Psychology* (6th ed.). Boston: Allyn & Bacon.

Leikin, S. L. (1989). Immunodeficiency virus infection, adolescents, and the institutional review board. *Journal of Adolescent Health Care, 10,* 500–505.

Leikin, S. L. (1993). Minors' assent, consent, or dissent to medical research. *IRB: A Review of Human Subjects Research, 15,* 1–7.

Levine, C., Dubler, N. N., & Levine, R. J. (1991). Building a new consensus: Ethical principles and policies for clinical research on HIV/AIDS. *IRB: A Review of Human Subjects Research, 13,* 1–17.

Lindsay, R. C., & Holden, R. R. (1987). The introductory psychology subject pool in Canadian universities. *Canadian Psychology, 28,* 45–52.

Long, H. B. (1982). Analysis of research concerning free and reduced tuition programs for senior citizens. *Educational Gerontology, 8,* 575–584.

Macklin, R. (1989). The paradoxical case of payment as benefit to research subjects. *IRB: A Review of Human Subjects Research, 11,* 1–3.

Mahler, D. M. (1986). When to obtain informed consent in behavioral research: A study of mother–infant bonding. *IRB: A Review of Human Subjects Research, 8,* 7–11.

Mammel, K. A., & Kaplan, D. W. (1995). Research consent of adolescent minors and institutional review boards. *Journal of Adolescent Health, 17,* 323–330.

Marshall, E. (1986). Does the moral philosophy of the Belmont Report rest on a mistake? *IRB: A Review of Human Subjects Research, 8,* 5–6.

Marvin, G. (1985). Evaluation research: Why a formal ethics review is needed. *Journal of Applied Social Sciences, 9,* 119–135.

McCord, D. M. (1991). Ethics-sensitive management of the university human subject pool. *American Psychologist, 46,* 151.

Megargee, E. I. (1995). Assessment research in correctional settings: Methodological issues and practical problems. *Psychological Assessment, 7,* 359–366.

Meinert, C. L. (1998). Masked monitoring in clinical trials: Blind stupidity? *New England Journal of Medicine, 338,* 1381–1382.

Meslin, E. M. (1990). Protecting human subjects from harm through improved risk judgments. *IRB: A Review of Human Subjects Research, 12,* 7–10.

Meyers, K., & Dunton, A. W. (1988). Applying "an ethical framework" to a proposed HIV antibody screening program. *IRB: A Review of Human Subjects Research, 10,* 6–8.

Miller, A. (1981). A survey of introductory psychology subject pool practices among leading universities. *Teaching of Psychology, 8,* 211–213.

Miller, F. G., & Rosenstein, D. L. (1997). Psychiatric symptom-provoking studies: An ethical appraisal. *Biological Psychiatry, 42,* 403–409.

Mordock, J. B. (1995). Institutional review boards in applied settings: Their role in judgments of quality and consumer protection. *Psychological Science, 6,* 320–321.

Murray, T. H. (1984). "The behavior of nonpsychologists on research review committees": Comment. *American Psychologist, 39,* 812–813.

National Commission for the Protection of Human Subjects of Biomedical and Behavioral Research. (1979). *The Belmont Report: Ethical Principles and Guidelines for the Protection of Human Subjects of Research.* Washington, DC: National Institutes of Health.

Newton, L. H. (1984). Agreement to participate in research: Is that a promise? *IRB: A Review of Human Subjects Research, 6,* 7–9.

Novick, A. (1984). At risk for AIDS: Confidentiality in research and surveillance. *IRB: A Review of Human Subjects Research, 6,* 10–11.

Office of Protection From Research Risks (OPRR). (1993). *Protecting human research subjects: Institutional review board guidebook.* Washington, DC: National Institutes of Health.

Orr, R. D. (1996). Guidelines for the use of placebo controls in clinical trials of psychopharmacologic agents. *Psychiatric Services, 47,* 1262–1264.

Ortega, R., & Dal-Re, R. (1995). Clinical trials committees: How long is the protocol review and approval process in Spain? A prospective study. *IRB: A Review of Human Subjects Research, 17,* 6–9.

Parker, L. S., & Lidz, C. W. (1994). Familial coercion to participate in genetic family studies: Is there cause for IRB intervention? *IRB: A Review of Human Subjects Research, 16,* 6–12.

Pattullo, E. L. (1987). Exemption from review, not informed consent. *IRB: A Review of Human Subjects Research, 9,* 6–8.

Perry, S. W. (1987). Pharmacological and psychological research on AIDS: Some ethical considerations. *IRB: A Review of Human Subjects Research, 9,* 8–10.

Peterson, B. T., Clancy, S. J., Champion, K., & McLarty, J. W. (1992). Improving readability of consent forms: What the computers may not tell you. *IRB: A Review of Human Subjects Research, 14,* 6–8.

Phillips, S. R. (1994). Asking the sensitive question: The ethics of survey research and teen sex. *IRB: A Review of Human Subjects Research, 16,* 1–7.

Pinals, D. A., Malhotra, A. K., Breier, A., & Pickar, D. (1998). Informed consent in schizophrenia research. *Psychiatric Services, 49,* 244.

Porter, J. P. (1986). What are the ideal characteristics of unaffiliated/nonscientist IRB members? *IRB: A Review of Human Subjects Research, 8,* 1–6.

Porter, J. P. (1987). How unaffiliated/nonscientist members of institutional review boards see their roles. *IRB: A Review of Human Subjects Research, 9,* 1–6.

Porter, J. P. (1991). The federal policy on the protection of human subjects. *IRB: A Review of Human Subjects Research, 13,* 8–9.

Porter, J. P. (1995). "Guidelines for adolescent participation in research: Current realities and possible resolutions": Reply. *IRB: A Review of Human Subjects Research, 17,* 10.

Porter, J. P., Glass, M. J., & Koff, W. C. (1989). Ethical considerations in AIDS vaccine testing. *IRB: A Review of Human Subjects Research, 11,* 1–4.

Powers, M. (1993). Publication–related risks to privacy: Ethical implications of pedigree studies. *IRB: A Review of Human Subjects Research*, 15, 7–11.

Prentice, E. D., Antonson, D. L., Leibrock, L. G., Kelso, T. K., & Sears, T. D. (1993). IRB review of a phase II randomized clinical trial involving incompetent patients suffering from severe closed head injury. *IRB: A Review of Human Subjects Research*, 15, 1–7.

Prentice, E. D., Reitemeier, P. J., Antonson, D. L., Kelso, T. K., & Jameton, A. (1993). Bill of rights for research subjects. *IRB: A Review of Human Subjects Research*, 15, 7–9.

Reese, H. W., & Fremouw, W. J. (1984). Normal and normative ethics in behavioral sciences. *American Psychologist*, 39, 863–876.

Reilly, P. R. (1991). Reviewing proposals to study biological correlates of criminality. *IRB: A Review of Human Subjects Research*, 13, 8–9.

Reiser, S. J., & Knudson, P. (1993). Protecting research subjects after consent: The case for the "research intermediary." *IRB: A Review of Human Subjects Research*, 15, 10–11.

Roberts, F. D., Newcomb, P. A., & Fost, N. (1993). Perceived risks of participation in an epidemiologic study. *IRB: A Review of Human Subjects Research*, 15, 8–10.

Rogers, A. S., D'Angelo, L., & Futterman, D. (1994). Guidelines for adolescent participation in research: Current realities and possible resolutions. *IRB: A Review of Human Subjects Research*, 16, 1–6.

Rosenthal, R. (1995). Ethical issues in psychological science: Risk, consent, and scientific quality. *Psychological Science*, 6, 322–323.

Rosnow, R. L., Rotheram-Borus, M. J., Ceci, S. J., Blanck, P. D., & Koocher, G. P. (1993). *American Psychologist*, 48, 821–826.

Schmidt, L. D., & Meara, N. M. (1996). Applying for approval to conduct research with human participants. In F. T. L. Leong, J. T. Austin, et al. (Eds.), *The psychology research handbook: A guide for graduate students and research assistants*. Thousand Oaks, CA: Sage.

Schreier, B. A., & Stadler, H. A. (1992). Perspectives of research participants, psychologist investigators, and institutional review boards. *Perceptual & Motor Skills*, 74, Special Issue.

Scott-Jones, D. (1994). Ethical issues in reporting and referring in research with low-income minority children. *Ethics & Behavior*, 4, 97–108.

Shamoo, A. E. (Ed.). (1997). *Ethics in neurobiological research with human subjects: The Baltimore conference on ethics*. India: Gordon and Breach Science.

Shimkin, M. B., Guttentag, O. E., Kidd, A. M., & Johnson, W. H. (1953). The problem of experimentation on human beings. *Science*, 117, 205–215.

Shimm, D. S., & Spece, R. G. (1992). Rate of refusal to participate in clinical trials. *IRB: A Review of Human Subjects Research*, 14, 7–9.

Sieber, J. E. (1989a). Sharing scientific data: I. New problems for IRBs. *IRB: A Review of Human Subjects Research*, 11, 4–7.

Sieber, J. E. (1989b). On studying the powerful (or fearing to do so): A vital role for IRBs. *IRB: A Review of Human Subjects Research, 11*, 1–6.

Sieber, J. E. (1992). *Planning ethically responsible research: A guide for students and internal review boards.* Newbury Park, CA: Sage.

Sieber, J. E. (1993). Ethical considerations in planning and conducting research on human subjects. *Academic Medicine, 68*, S9–S13.

Sieber, J. E. (1994a). Issues presented by mandatory reporting requirements to researchers of child abuse and neglect. *Ethics & Behavior, 4*, 1–22.

Sieber, J. E. (1994b). Will the new code help researchers to be more ethical? *Professional Psychology: Research & Practice, 49*, 369–375.

Sieber, J. E., & Saks, M. J. (1989). A census of subject pool characteristics and policies. *American Psychologist, 44*, 1053–1061.

Silva, M. C., & Sorrell, J. M. (1988). Enhancing comprehension of information for informed consent: A review of empirical research. *IRB: A Review of Human Subjects Research, 10*, 1–5.

Smith, M. A., & Leigh, B. (1997). Virtual subjects: Using the Internet as an alternative source of subjects and research environment. *Behavior Research Methods, Instruments, & Computers, 29*, 496–505.

Spilker, B. (1992). Methods of assessing and improving patient compliance in clinical trials. *IRB: A Review of Human Subjects Research, 14*, 1–6.

Stuart, R. B. (1978). Protection of the right to informed consent to participate in research. *Behavior Therapy, 9*, 73–82.

Taub, H. A. (1986). Comprehension of informed consent in research: Issues and directions for future study. *IRB: A Review of Human Subjects Research, 8*, 7–10.

Taube, D. O., & Burkhardt, S. (1997). Ethical and legal risks associated with archival research. *Ethics & Behavior, 7*, 59–67.

Theut, S. K., & Kohrman, A. F. (1990). Ethical issues in research in child psychiatry. In S. I. Deutsch, Wiezman, A., et al. (Eds.), *Application of basic neuroscience to child psychiatry* (pp. 383–389). New York: Plenum Press.

Treadway, J. T., & Rossi, R. B. (1977). An ethical review board: Its structure, function and province. *Mental Retardation, 15*, 28–29.

Trials of War Criminals Before the Nuremberg Military Tribunals Under Control Council Law No. 10. (1949). *Nuremberg Code* (Vol. 2, pp. 181–182). Washington, DC: U.S. Government Printing Office.

Tuthill, K. A. (1997). Human experimentation: Promoting patient autonomy through informed consent. *Journal of Legal Medicine, 18*, 221–250.

Waggoner, W. C., & Mayo, D. M. (1995). Who understands? A survey of 25 words or phrases commonly used in proposed clinical research consent forms. *IRB: A Review of Human Subjects Research, 17*, 6–9.

White, L. K., & Morse, L. A. (1988). Behavior modification in institutions: The development of legal protections of patients' rights. *Behavioral Residential Treatment, 3*, 287–314.

Wieman, H. N. (1922). The unique in human behaviar [sic]. *Psychological Review, 29*, 414–425.

Williams, J. G., & Ouren, L. H. (1976). Experimenting on humans. *Bulletin of the British Psychological Society, 29*, 334–338.

Williams, P. C. (1984). Success in spite of failure: Why IRBs falter in reviewing risks and benefits. *IRB: A Review of Human Subjects Research, 6*, 1–4.

World Medical Assembly. (1964). *Declaration of Helsinki.* Helsinki, Finland: 18th World Medical Assembly.

Young, D. R., Hooker, D. T., & Freeberg, F. E. (1990). Informed consent documents: Increasing comprehension by reducing reading level. *IRB: A Review of Human Subjects Research, 12*, 1–5.

Young, S. N. (1998). Risks in research: From the Nuremberg Code to the Tri-Council Code: Implications for clinical trials of psychotropic drugs. *Journal of Psychiatry & Neuroscience, 23*, 149–155.

I

Human Subject Research From a Departmental Perspective

This first section addresses issues related to developing and managing a departmental subject pool (DSP). The concerns that are treated are those incident to the founding and successful day to day operation of a DSP. The importance of implementing appropriate procedures and policies at the time a DSP is established cannot be overemphasized. Moreover, knowing what issues are likely to arise after the DSP has begun and how to cope with those issues are vital to the ethical and competent management of a DSP.

Chapter 1 provides the results of a national survey of DSP practices in undergraduate-only departments. It offers information about the prevalence of DSPs and Institutional Review Boards (IRBs) in public and private institutions, types of incentives for and alternatives to participation in DSPs, and ways that the educational value of the experience is assessed.

Chapter 2 presents a detailed discussion of DSP ethics, including informed consent, alternatives to DSP participation, follow-up assessments of how participants were treated and the educational benefits of participation, and all parties for whom DSP procedures should be developed and why.

1

Subject Pool Policies in Undergraduate-Only Departments: Results From a Nationwide Survey

R. Eric Landrum and Garvin Chastain

Psychology has long relied on and been committed to empirical research. Indeed, empiricism is the foundation and hallmark of the discipline. Psychologists' understanding of human behavior has come largely from the study of humans—oftentimes student recruits from a college or university human subject pool (HSP). Although the estimates vary (see Kulich, Seldon, Richardson, & Servies, 1978), it seems clear that the great majority of results of human studies published in the literature has come from subject pool participants. Given the dual responsibility of reliance on this resource and the protection of human subjects, it seems prudent to understand in better detail the policies and procedures that lead to the availability of this resource–opportunity, and also to understand how the HSP policies and procedures may affect the outcomes of the studies conducted.

In reviewing the literature, four themes emerge that are related to the topic of HSP practices: (a) student attitudes about research participation, (b) research concerning student participation and time of semester, (c) how Institutional Review Board (IRB) regulations affect research, and (d) experimenter responsibility in research. Given psychology's dependence on subject pool participants, there seems to be relatively little research conducted to examine these issues. Following the review, we present some of our empirical research on the topic.

Student Attitudes About Research Participation

One area of research involves studies of the attitudes of college student participants in the human subject pool. Britton (1979), in a survey of students, found that although politeness, adequate explanations, and personal comfort provided by the experimenter were rated highly on the scale used, the educational value of the research experience was rated somewhat lower. Miller, in a study of top research universities, concluded that "little has been done to provide evidence that experimental participation is a valuable pedagogical device" (1981, p. 213). Coulter (1986) also reported on student complaints about research and the researchers' lack of interest in debriefing and educating student participants.

These findings provoke serious questions about the participative value of research. On the other hand, many have demonstrated some of the positive outcomes of subject pool participation. Holmes (1967) found that more experienced participants tended to see experiments as scientifically valuable, which increased their levels of cooperation. Leak (1981) found that students view the research experience positively. Nimmer and Handelsman (1992) found that students were more positive toward research participation when it was semivoluntary and did not require an inordinate time commitment. Landrum and Chastain (1995) found that students reported that their participation in experiments helped them to learn about psychology and to better understand the research process.

Although the results are mixed, evidence does seem to support the conclusion that if done appropriately, research can be of pedagogical value to students. Study results may vary as a result of the different methods used to assess student opinion. Mann (1995) found in her research with informed consent that long forms, although thorough, are not well-understood by research participants: Signing the informed consent without understanding it is not providing informed consent. Mann found that few participants understand what to do or what procedures to follow if they have a complaint about the experiment or suffer adverse effects from it.

Time of Semester and Student Participation

There have been a handful of studies that have examined the time during a semester that a student participates in a study (usually *early* or *late*) to determine whether students perform differently at different times. Underwood, Schwenn, and Keppel (1964) found no evidence of significant differences between early and late participants' performance on a verbal learning task. Similarly, Langston, Ohnesorge, Kruley, and Haase (1994) found no significant time-of-semester differences in signal detection or text comprehension tasks. However, Holden and Reddon (1987) found that personality characteristics do differ on some dimensions between early- and late-semester participants. Late-semester male participants scored as less socially responsible than early-semester male participants, and late-semester participants of both genders demonstrated higher exhibitionistic and playful characteristics compared to early-semester participants. Holmes (1967) found that students' first research experience influenced their perceptions of later research experiences. The more experienced participants valued scientific research more, tried harder to cooperate, and did not try as hard to "figure out" the experiment.

How IRB Regulations Affect Research

When subject pools are used at universities that are required to have an IRB (usually because the university receives federal funding), subject pools are inextricably linked to IRBs. Some of the scholarly materials that address subject pool issues also address IRB concerns. Adair, Dushenko, and Lindsay (1985) lamented the fact that ethical practices are seldom reported in published research (e.g., describing what participants are told). In addition, they found that whereas the American Psychological Association (APA) has adopted restrictive ethical guidelines limiting the use of deception in research, this does not seem to have an impact on the use of deception. It may be that Adair et al. (1985) expected stricter guidelines to reduce deceptive research, or to dissuade researchers from using deception.

In studying how IRBs and human subjects committees make decisions on proposals, Ceci, Peters, and Plotkin (1985) submitted hypothetical proposals to IRBs, with proposals on sensitive and nonsensitive topics. Sensitive proposals were for studying corporate hiring practices and included discrimination or reverse discrimination based on race or gender. Nonsensitive proposals were methodologically identical except discrimination was based on height or weight. Socially sensitive proposals were twice as likely to be rejected by IRBs, and the more common reason given by IRBs was methodological.

In examining the practices of IRBs, Rosnow, Rotheram-Borus, Ceci, Blanck, and Koocher (1993) studied the changing role of IRBs and addressed two important questions: (a) should IRBs be involved in the evaluation of whether the research has scientific merit, and (b) should rules and regulations be strictly followed in the face of dramatically changing research scenarios? Their recommendation to IRBs was to stay abreast of emerging issues, in part by assessing risk–benefit ratios within the confines of their charge, and also by improving the training and decision-making processes used by IRB members such as reviewing research scenarios from a casebook. An excellent resource in this regard is available, edited by Bersoff (1995), called *Ethical Conflicts in Psychology*.

Experimenter Responsibility in Research

A fourth area of concern that emerges regarding subject pool and related research issues is the responsibility of the experimenter in the conduct of research. This typically emerges as an issue of balance—between the costs of the research to participants versus the benefits of the research to psychology and society, and also a balance between the ethical quality and the scientific quality of research. Rosenthal (1994) makes the point that research of higher scientific quality is likely to be more ethically defensible. That is, "the lower the quality of the research, the less justified we are ethically to waste research participants' time, funding agencies' money, and journals' space" (p. 127). The issue of balance between cost versus benefit has been raised. Kimmel (1979) reported on ethical violations and the consequences of such actions, and Palij (1988) and Fisher and Fyrberg (1995) have discussed the cost versus benefit trade-off as part of an experimenter's responsibility in research.

Rosenthal (1994) addressed the balance between scientific quality of research and the ethical quality of research, and concluded that the two are not independent. By examining the issues surrounding the conduct, analysis, and reporting of psychological research, he noted that improvements in one area (scientific quality) can lead to improvements in other areas (ethical quality). Another conclusion that can be drawn from this relationship between scientific quality and ethical quality is that IRBs might be involved in the judgment of methodological adequacy, perhaps only to the extent of ensuring that the research is not a waste of participants' time.

Toward Our Research

The seminal article to date concerning subject pool policies and procedures is by Sieber and Saks (1989). In a national survey of psychology departments with graduate programs, 74.0% reported having subject pools. Of those with subject pools, 60.6% were from doctoral programs. Only 11.0% of graduate departments reported having completely voluntary subject pools. To avoid coercing student participation, other alternatives are frequently made available. Educational value, although of interest to Sieber and Saks, was not addressed directly in their survey of graduate departments.

Our focus is on undergraduate departments of psychology (those offering a 4-year baccalaureate degree in psychology or a related field). Because of the nature of graduate training, it seems reasonable that a great deal of research (and use of subject pools) is generated through graduate faculty and graduate students. It also appears that in some areas a greater emphasis on research at the undergraduate level is taking place (for example, academic organizations such as the National Council for Undergraduate Research and the Council for Undergraduate Research that advocate such research). We are interested in many of the issues Sieber and Saks (1989) pursued with graduate institutions, including (a) the prevalence of subject pools; (b) the policies and requirements of subjects pools—in other words, coerciveness; (c) the assessment of educational value of subject pool participation for students; and (d) the cataloging of the most common subject pool practices as well as identifying unique and interesting approaches.

Method

Participants

We chose to survey departments with only an undergraduate program in psychology because there seems to be some indication of a general increase in research productivity at undergraduate institutions (based on informal conversations with colleagues at conferences), and because our own university has a psychology department without a graduate program.

The names and address labels for undergraduate-only psychology departments in the United States were obtained from APA's Office of Demographic, Employment, and Educational

Research (ODEER). ODEER identified 1238 departments that met our criteria. All 1238 departments were surveyed.

Materials

We developed a two-page survey and mailed it to all potential participants. Surveys were coded in a fashion that allowed respondents and nonrespondents to be identified and tracked. Survey respondents were aware of this process. Some of the questions were included to ascertain information similar to other surveys. We also included Miller's (1981) questions concerning how subjects are solicited and how the educational value of the subject pool experience is evaluated. A number of university- and departmental-type demographic questions were also asked. These questions, accompanied by descriptive statistics, can be found in Table 1-1.

Procedure

The survey package included the two-page survey (the front and back of one piece of paper) and a self-addressed, business-reply return mail envelope. Instructions for completing the survey were included on the survey form and not in a separate cover letter. Approximately 6 weeks after the surveys were sent, a follow-up postcard was mailed to all nonrespondents.

We received 590 of 1238 surveys (47.6%). Given the nature of mail survey research, bulk-rate mail, and the difficulty in reaching very busy people, we were pleased with that response rate and believed that we hit a nerve with our undergraduate-only counterpart institutions. Of the 590 surveys returned, 478 (81.0%) provided usable responses. Of the 112 unusable responses, 85.7% of those were from departments reporting that they have a graduate program. Some departments had recently added graduate programs, and some of the labels were provided in error. All further data analyses were based on usable responses from undergraduate-only departments. Thus the corrected response rate was 41.9% (478 out of 1,142).

Table 1-1

Descriptive Statistics on Survey Questions: Overall and Public Versus Private Institution

Question	Overall	Type of school		N
		Public	Private	
Total number of schools contacted	1238	271	967	
Undergraduate schools' and number responding	1142	135	340	
University enrollment	2339.97	3799.85	1771.60	466
	(3632.04)	(3400.60)	(3574.54)	
Number of full-time faculty	5.86	7.21	5.33	477
	(11.00)	(10.48)	(11.21)	
Number of part-time/adjunct faculty	3.82	3.47	3.97	464
	(8.81)	(4.55)	(10.03)	
Number of majors	106.95	163.29	85.22	471
	(113.79)	(166.61)	(73.93)	
Number of active researchers in psychology department	3.13	4.64	2.51	463
	(5.45)	(9.00)	(2.85)	
Does department offer a bachelor's degree in psychology?[a]	86.9%	81.5%	89.0%	475
If yes, how many awarded per year?	27.96	38.91	24.16	418
	(24.49)	(35.09)	(19.91)	
Total annual enrollment in general introductory psychology	344.00	624.91	236.92	463
	(394.92)	(610.92)	(181.85)	
Does your institution have an institutional review board?[a]	55.5%	71.6%	48.7%	474
Does your department have a human subjects pool?[a]	32.7%	40.5%	29.7%	471
How are subjects solicited?[b]				455

Totally volunteer	34.7%	28.7%
Extra credit	18.9%	16.2%
Extra credit with other options to earn same credit	24.8%	28.7%
Requirement	3.3%	4.4%
Requirement with other options to fulfill requirement	14.1%	19.8%
Other	4.2%	2.2%
How do you assess the educational value of the subject pool		337
Experience for students?[b]		
Knowledge is tested	4.5%	4.2%
Student's perception of value is assessed	13.0%	13.2%
Students complete experiment-associated assignment	11.9%	10.2%
No assessment is done	62.9%	64.2%
Other	7.7%	8.1%

NOTE: Where appropriate, means are reported with standard deviations in parentheses.
[a]This number represents the percentage of participants answering *yes*.
[b]On these questions, participants were able to report more than one category. These percentages reflect the proportion of times the item was selected out of all possible selections, not the proportion of participants selecting that category. *N* reflects the total number of responses.

Results and Discussion

Prevalence of Subject Pools

For undergraduate psychology departments, how prevalent are subject pools currently? Overall, 32.7% of undergraduate departments report having a subject pool, compared to 74.0% of graduate psychology departments (Sieber & Saks, 1989). As noted in Table 1-1, 28.4% of the responses came from public colleges or universities, whereas 71.6% came from private colleges or universities. The 135 and 340 usable responses from public and private institutions, respectively, indicate that 49.8% of the public institutions and 35.1% of the private institutions responded to our survey request. Prevalence of subject pools does vary by type of institution, as public institutions are more likely to have a subject pool than private institutions—40.5% versus 29.7%, respectively (X^2 [1, N = 468] = 4.98, $p < .05$). It seems that subject pools are not as prevalent in undergraduate departments as they are in graduate departments, even when comparing current undergraduate data with older graduate data. In asking undergraduate departments about subject pools, we also asked about IRBs. Fifty-five percent of undergraduate psychology departments reported that their institution had an IRB, and 71.6% and 48.7% of the public and private universities, respectively, reported an IRB. This proportion of public institutions having IRBs is significantly higher than private institutions having IRBs (χ^2 [1, N = 471] = 20.46, $p < .001$).

We also examined the relationship between having an IRB and having an HSP. Of the undergraduate departments that have an HSP (154), 75.3% have an IRB; of the 317 schools that do not have an HSP, only 45.3% have an IRB. Having an HSP is significantly associated with having an IRB (χ^2 [1, N = 469] = 37.46, $p < .001$).

Coerciveness of Subject Pools

In Sieber and Saks's (1989) treatment of coercion, they examined the ways that departments implement their guidelines. For example, they looked at information published in university catalogs and course syllabi. They also reported on the alternatives to research participation reported by graduate departments, which included writing a paper (62.7% departments reported offering this option), giving extra homework or quiz (8.8%), watching a movie or demonstration (8.0%), or some other alternative (31.0%). We chose to use the same tactic as Miller (1981), and asked departments to indicate how participants are solicited. The available options as answers to this question are presented in Table 1-1. At the undergraduate level, the modal method for soliciting is totally volunteer (34.7%), followed by extra credit with other options to obtain same credit (24.8%) and just extra credit (18.9%). These preferences clearly differ from those used by top research universities as reported by Miller (1981). Miller found that 58.6% of those universities based participation on a requirement, with other options to satisfy that requirement. In our study of undergraduate departments, the frequency of methods used by departments did differ just marginally between public and private institutions (χ^2 [5, N = 452] = 10.94, p = .052).

Educational Value

A primary justification for the use of subject pools is for the educational value the research experience can provide to the undergraduate student (Landrum & Chastain, 1995). This experience tends to differ dramatically from the typical classroom-instruction type of learning, giving students a chance to experience psychology hands-on (e.g., we encourage our general psychology students to ask their experimenters about the independent and dependent variables in the study). Sieber and Saks (1989) found it difficult to determine educational value because they examined only the protocols and procedures used by graduate departments. We again chose the approach of Miller (1981), and we asked undergraduate departments how they assessed the educational value of the subject pool experience for students. As seen in Table 1-1, the most frequent method of assessing value is not to assess it at all (62.9%), compared to Miller's (1981) 77.1% not assessing it at all for top research universities. When assessment is done, the most common technique is to assess the student's perception of value, and the frequency of use of this assessment technique does not differ depending on public or private institution (χ^2 [4, N = 333] = 2.46, n.s.).

Subject Pool Protocols

We asked undergraduate departments to enclose a copy of their HSP guidelines/protocol, and 79 did so (29.8% overall). We also asked them to explain, if they did not want to send them, why they did not want to. "The department does not have formal guidelines, hence they cannot be sent" was reported by 90.7%, whereas 9.3% indicated that they had such guidelines but chose not to share them (respondents did not indicate why they chose not to include their guidelines). A content analysis of the protocols focused on three areas: general themes that emerge in subject pool operations, alternative options to research participation, and identification of the unique and interesting approaches and perspectives used by undergraduate departments. Some of these results have been previously presented (Davis, Chastain, & Landrum, 1996).

In examining the protocols collected, four themes emerged that seem to be relatively consistent across human subject pool policies and procedures. Subject pool guidelines typically state the amount of time required of students for participation, how much credit students gain by participating or lose by not participating, the consequences of noncompliance or not showing up for the research appointment, and the alternative forms of research credit available to students. Note that in some cases, however, some of this does not apply. If the subject pool participants are all volunteers, then there would not be a discussion of how much credit one loses by not participating. In examining these protocols, it is clear that each department places its institutional imprint on the policies and procedures used.

In Sieber and Saks's (1989) report of graduate departments, they commented on the lack of apparent variety of alternatives students could pursue to fulfill a research requirement. It appears that the undergraduate departments in our study employ a wider variety of approaches. The alternative options used to fulfill research participation requirements include (a) writing a paper reviewing a journal article; (b) observing an experimental session and writing a brief paper describing the experiment; (c) conducting a case study using yourself as a participant in some sort of simulation; (d) watching a videotape related to general psychology and participating afterward in a discussion led by a laboratory assistant; (e) attending a research colloquium, presentation, or "brown bag" lecture sponsored by the psychology department; (f) attending student presentation sessions of research from upper-division psychology courses; and (g) negotiating an individualized research participation project proposed by the student and approved by the instructor. This list should prove to be valuable to those who are looking to expand the number of ways students can fulfill research experience requirements (or to those planning to create a subject pool).

Although commonalties certainly emerged across the HSP protocols, there were also a number of unique and interesting discoveries made about the various processes used around the country. For example, some departments mandate that students provide feedback about the research experience and offer credit for the feedback in addition to credit for completing the research experience (some require students to write about the experience after participating). Other departments are cautious and strict about the nature of the debriefing offered to students, differentiating between debriefing, dehoaxing, and desensitization. Some departments require "extreme" debriefing, even for innocuous studies with no risk. Others require students to sign a contract indicating that they will not discuss the hypothesis of the experiment with other students, and some HSPs require that results of the study must either be posted or mailed to participants. Some departments, usually in private institutions, require that the studies conducted with the subject pool participants be consistent with the school's religious or philosophical orientation. Again, these types of perspectives are invaluable for those wishing to review how their human subject pool operates or for those contemplating creating a subject pool. Of those departments that did not have a subject pool (67.3%), 34 universities (12.3%) indicated that they plan to have a subject pool in the future. The resources made available in this volume should be useful for those continuing and improving subject pool practices as well as for those implementing a new subject pool.

Predicting the Presence of HSPs and IRBs

Examining these relationships led us to think about the institutional characteristics that might predict whether or not an institution has an HSP or an IRB. Considering HSPs, we examined the relationship between the demographic characteristics reported from the survey and the presence or absence of an HSP. The analyses examined the multivariate effects by regressing HSP status (exists or does not exist) onto the demographic characteristics. Together, the predictors accounted for 19.5% of the variance in HSP status ($F[10, 395] = 9.58, p < .001$).

Further examination revealed significant unique effects for the institutional characteristics of number of part-time faculty ($b = -0.147, t = -2.46, p < .05$), number of active researchers in the department ($b = 0.190, t = 3.69, p < .001$), whether or not the department grants a bachelor's degree in psychology ($b = 0.149, t = 2.96, p < .01$), and whether or not the institution has an IRB ($b = 0.145, t = 2.89, p < .01$).

Undergraduate departments of psychology tend to have human subject pools when the number of part-time faculty is small and when the department has a higher number of active researchers. Also, HSPs are more likely when the department is degree-granting and when the institution has an IRB. These variables seem to indicate that HSPs are evident when there is high enough research activity to warrant it (evidenced by higher number of active researchers and an IRB presence) and when departments have, perhaps, a longer term commitment to and more resources for their students (degree-granting and fewer part-time faculty).

What predicts the presence of an IRB? Similar regression analyses were conducted between the demographic characteristics available and IRB status *(present, not present)*. Together, the predictors accounted for 20.4% of the variance in IRB status ($F[10, 395] = 10.11, p < .001$). Further examination yielded significant unique effects for the institutional characteristics of university enrollment ($b = 0.148, t = 2.27, p < .05$), number of full-time faculty ($b = 0.129, t = 2.35, p < .05$), whether or not the department grants the bachelor's degree in psychology ($b = 0.128, t = 2.56, p < .05$), and whether the institution has an HSP ($b = 0.143, t = 2.89, p < .01$).

Size and research activity seem to be components of whether or not an institution has an IRB, as seen by the regression outcomes with university enrollments and number of full-time faculty. Degree-granting status is a significant predictor of both HSPs and IRBs, and the presence of an IRB is a significant predictor of an HSP, and vice versa. IRBs are evident when size of institution and size of faculty warrant it, and the institution has a longer term commitment to students and research, as seen by the presence of degree-granting status and an HSP.

Conclusion

Research in this area has focused on four issues: student attitudes about participation in research projects, the time of semester students participate in research, IRB regulations, and experimenter responsibility in research. Of those responding to a national survey, 32.7% of undergraduate institutions responded that they have a subject pool, and public universities are more likely to have a subject pool (40.5%) than private institutions (29.7%). We also found that 55.5% of the undergraduate psychology departments have an IRB, but the IRBs are more prevalent at public (71.6%) than private (48.7%) institutions. The modal technique for recruiting participants is by using a totally volunteer subject pool (34.7%), followed by using extra credit with other options to obtain credit (24.8%), with more than half of the responding departments (62.9%) not assessing the educational value of the subject's research experience. We suggest that this is an important component of the process, and we have recommended a method for assessment (Landrum & Chastain, 1995). Other educational options for students who choose not to participate in research include writing a paper, observing an experiment, conducting a case study, watching a videotape, attending a colloquium, attending a conference, or designing a project.

On the whole, it does seem that undergraduate departments of psychology differ in many respects from graduate departments in terms of both HSPs and IRBs. Even among undergraduate departments, there is a great deal of variability with respect to the type and size of school and how HSPs and IRBs operate, and even whether they are present or not. More scholarly research needs to be conducted in these areas. If we consider the number of participant-hours students provide to researchers nationwide, it seems clear that we have an obligation to ensure that the experience is educational, nonstressful, and occurs without coercion. To do anything less would be unethical.

References

Adair, J. G., Dushenko, T. W., & Lindsay, R. C. L. (1985). Ethical regulations and their impact on research practice. *American Psychologist, 40,* 59–72.

American Psychological Association. (1979). *Ethical standards of psychologists.* Washington, DC: Author.

American Psychological Association. (1981). Ethical principles of psychologists. *American Psychologist, 36,* 633–638.

American Psychological Association. (1990). Ethical principles of psychologists (Amended June 2, 1989). *American Psychologist, 45,* 390–395.

American Psychological Association. (1992). *APA ethics code.* Washington, DC: Author.

Bersoff, D. N. (Ed.). (1995). *Ethical conflicts in psychology.* Washington, DC: American Psychological Association.

Britton, B. K. (1979). Ethical and educational aspects of participating as a subject in psychology experiments. *Teaching of Psychology, 6*, 195–198.

Ceci, S. J., Peters, D., & Plotkin, J. (1985). Human subjects review, personal values, and the regulation of social science research. *American Psychologist, 40*, 994–1002.

Coulter, X. (1986). Academic value of research participation by undergraduates. *American Psychologist, 41*, 317.

Davis, R., Chastain, G., & Landrum, R. E. (1996, May). *Protocols of department subject pools: A national sample.* Paper presented at the Midwestern Psychological Association, Chicago.

Fisher, C. B., & Fyrberg, D. (1995). Participant partners: College students weigh the costs and benefits of deceptive research. In D. N. Bersoff (Ed.), *Ethical conflicts in psychology.* Washington, DC: American Psychological Association.

Holden, R. R., & Reddon, J. R. (1987). Temporal personality variations among participants from a university subject pool. *Psychological Reports, 60*, 1247–1254.

Holmes, D. S. (1967). Amount of experience in experiments as a determinant of performance in later experiments. *Journal of Personality and Social Psychology, 7*, 403–407.

Kimmel, A. J. (1979). Ethics and human subjects research: A delicate balance. *American Psychologist, 34*, 633–635.

Kulich, R. J., Seldon, J. W., Richardson, K., & Servies, S. (1978, May). *Frequency of employing undergraduate samples in psychological research and subject reaction to forced participation.* Paper presented at the Midwestern Psychological Association, Chicago.

Landrum, R. E., & Chastain, G. (1995). Experiment spot-checks: A method for assessing the educational value of undergraduate participation in research. *IRB: A Review of Human Subjects Research, 17*, 4–6.

Langston, W., Ohnesorge, C., Kruley, P., & Hasse, S. J. (1994). Changes in subject performance during the semester: An empirical investigation. *Psychonomic Bulletin & Review, 1*, 258–263.

Leak, G. K. (1981). Student perception of coercion and value from participation in psychological research. *Teaching of Psychology, 8*, 147–149.

Miller, A. (1981). A survey of introductory psychology subject pool practices among leading universities. *Teaching of Psychology, 8*, 211–213.

Nimmer, J. G., & Handelsman, M. M. (1992). Effects of subject pool policy on student attitudes toward psychology and psychological research. *Teaching of Psychology, 19*, 141–144.

Palij, M. (1988). What happens to the unwanted subject? Comment on the value of undergraduate participation in research. *American Psychologist, 43*, 404–405.

Rosenthal, R. (1994). Science and ethics in conducting, analyzing, and reporting psychological research. *Psychological Science, 5*, 127–134.

Rosnow, R. L., Rotheram-Borus, M. J., Ceci, S. J., Blanck, P. D., & Koocher,

G. P. (1993). The Institutional Review Board as a mirror of scientific and ethical standards. *American Psychologist, 48,* 821–826.

Sieber, J. E., & Saks, M. J. (1989). A census of subject pool characteristics and policies. *American Psychologist, 44,* 1053–1061.

Underwood, B. J., Schwenn, E., & Keppel, G. (1964). Verbal learning as related to point of time in the school term. *Journal of Verbal Learning and Verbal Behavior, 3,* 222–225.

2

What Makes a Subject Pool (Un)ethical?

Joan E. Sieber

Subject pools—those course requirements that conveniently provide research subjects to faculty and advanced students—came about decades before researchers felt much concern for legal and ethical issues connected with human research. In today's legal climate, how could a course requirement that students participate in research be permissible? Subject pools are like aspirin, which would never pass today's Food and Drug Administration requirements. Subject pools have been "grandfathered" in. But unlike aspirin, most subject pool practices have been modified over the years to comply, or nearly comply, with current standards of research

This chapter is based on research performed in collaboration with Michael J. Saks (Sieber & Saks, 1989) and on some of the outstanding subject pool policy statements that various departments of psychology graciously provided. I am grateful to Michael Saks for his productive initial collaboration, and to him and Eleanor Levine for their valuable comments on this manuscript.

The departments that created the outstanding materials paraphrased in this chapter gave their permission for such use. Anonymity was promised and identifiers were removed from the materials. I no longer know who provided these materials, and could not reveal that information even if I did know. My respect and appreciation of the creators of these materials is immense.

practice. This chapter seeks to discover how much they have been modified; what kinds of creative new administrative and education policies have been developed to bring subject pools into compliance with legal and ethical standards; what remains to be done to improve the ethics of subject pool practices; and whether any of this matters—in other words, are subject pools still prevalent enough today to make them worth our professional concern?

The Prevalence of Subject Pools

Much psychological research comes about through the use of undergraduate subject pools. In 1977, 73.2% of articles in the *Journal of Personality and Social Psychology (JPSP)* and 92.7% of the articles in the *Journal of Experimental Psychology: Perception* were reports of research involving subject pool participants (Kulich, Seldon, Richardson, & Servies, 1978). In 1980, 76% of the articles in *JPSP* reflected subject pool use, and in 1987, 74% of the articles in *JPSP* did so (Sieber, Iannuzzo, & Rodriguez, 1995). In a 1989 survey of all psychology departments in the United States that have graduate programs, it appeared that every department having much involvement with research had a subject pool. All of the departments having 45 faculty members or more reported having a subject pool, and of the smaller departments, 74% reported having a subject pool. In departments having subject pools, 93.4% recruit from introductory psychology courses, 35.4% from lower division courses, and 7.7% recruit from other sources as well (Sieber & Saks, 1989).

Having subject-pool requirements built into courses raises ethical questions. How voluntary is participation? Are subject pools administered in compliance with federal law governing research and with the APA's ethical code? For example, how can participation be voluntary (as required by law) and at the same time a requirement built into a lower division course? The standard justification for having subject pool requirements built into courses is that student participants receive educational benefits. But are the students who participate in subject pools actually receiving the educational benefits that purportedly flow from that experience?

Methodological issues also need to be considered. Invalid research is unethical. How valid is a sample drawn from a subject pool? To what populations can it be generalized? How contaminated are the data by the games that bored or disgruntled students play with experimenters?

The Implications for Departments of Psychology

If subject pools are conducted with ethical sensitivity, a win–win situation is created. Valid knowledge is generated, students have a worthwhile educational experience, and students develop an understanding of ethical practices in psychology. If subject pools are administered in a shoddy fashion, students are disrespected and grow cynical about science, perhaps to the point of sabotaging the research in which they participate. Worse, students fail to learn how to conduct research ethically for lack of adequate role models.

Subject pools do not operate in a vacuum within departments. They are an intellectual and moral extension of the way the rest of the department operates. Does the department invent new and better rules and procedures—ones that turn ethical conflicts into win–win situations? How can it create a professional culture that breathes life into these rules and procedures—gives them vitality and meaning so that they spring from each person's understanding of what it means to be ethical? Without such a culture, the rules and procedures become the embodiment of mindless bureaucracy.

How can subject pool practices reflect a professional culture of ethical sensitivity, and convey this sensitivity to students? How can other aspects of teaching, and of the psychology curriculum and related departmental activities, embody and teach ethical professional practices in psychology? These questions reach far beyond subject pools—into the classroom, and into the ethical mentoring of faculty and students. And they reach into the many venues in which researchers and clinicians work—communities, clinical settings, industry, schools, hospitals, and so on.

Many questions regarding possible careless and expedient practices that make subject pools unethical and creative management of subject pools that make them ethical were answered empirically by asking psychology department faculty about their subject pool practices. In this chapter, I discuss what we learned about current subject pool practices. I spell out some of the details of good practice (but mostly refer the reader to an archive of those details), and point to some sources of education, ethical guidance, leadership, and creative problem solving that are the intellectual and moral engine that powers these activities.

A Study of Subject Pool Practices

A survey (Sieber & Saks, 1989) was designed to reveal the nature and prevalence of exemplary, adequate, and poor subject pool practices, and also whether psychology departments are entirely candid about deficiencies in their subject pool practices. This chapter is based largely on the findings of that survey and on the exemplary policies and procedures that some respondents generously shared.

An Experiment Within a Survey

The candor of survey respondents cannot practically be assessed directly. But it is possible to determine whether (randomly assigned) anonymous respondents more frequently admit to questionable practices than their identified counterparts.

Half of our respondents were asked to indicate their name and the name of their university. The other half were to respond anonymously. Identified respondents were found to be as likely to admit illegal or unethical practices as anonymous respondents, but they gave lots of excuses for their actions, whereas the anonymous respondents did not. From this, we surmise that we hit a sensitive nerve. Those required to identify themselves apparently felt embarrassed and defensive when admitting dubious activities, and some few who were asked to identify themselves (and who indicated some poor practices) returned their survey without identifying themselves.

We invited respondents to send us their subject pool policy, which might expose their identity and practices. Only 19% of the anonymous respondents sent theirs, and some removed identifying information. A few of the respondents randomly assigned to the anonymous condition insisted on sending us their policies and procedures, and identifying themselves, contrary to our instructions—and not surprisingly, these were the ones with exemplary procedures. Among the identified respondents, 31% sent their policy and procedure documents, including some that raised minor ethical concerns. It appeared that those with impressive policies wished to show them to us and to identify themselves even if they were in the anonymous condition, and those required to identify themselves wanted to proffer something, anything that could put them in a good light. But most in the anonymous condition were content to keep their policies and identity from us.

What Makes for Poor Subject Pool Practices?

Noncompliance with Federal Law and APA Guidelines

Because subject pools have been around far longer than federal regulations or APA ethical guidelines governing human research, it could be that some subject pools have not updated their policies to reflect newer standards. Federal law requires an adequate review process to ensure risk–benefit assessment and compliance, informed consent, and voluntariness of participation. However, 11% of departments lack an explicit requirement of informed consent, and 29% lack a mandatory application policy for subject pool use. APA guidelines urge departments to announce subject pool requirements in the course catalog, but only 20.1% of respondents do so. At the first class meeting, 92% announce the requirement, 89% disclose how much participation is required, 85% mention the right to withdraw without penalty, 83% describe available alternatives to participation, 82% describe benefits of participation, 69% mention the researcher's obligation to be respectful, 56% discuss the complaint procedure, 46% provide information on any penalties or nonappearance, and 41% describe projects from which students may choose. Many departments that offer alternatives to participation do not include attractive alternatives such as a movie or demonstration (8%), requiring instead a paper (63%) or extra coursework and a quiz (9%). Without attractive alternatives, subject pool participation cannot be considered voluntary; rather, it is coercive. Only 8% of departments had a subject pool that is voluntary in the strictest sense— in other words, having no penalties for nonparticipation, no grades for participation, and no alternatives to participation.

Lack of Educational Value for Participants

Educational value is a major rationale for having subject pools. There should be an appropriate quid pro quo in which the student provides useful data and is repaid in kind—with interesting knowledge, respectfully conveyed, not with money or grades. Meaningless research experience would be chosen only as the lesser evil, which amounts to coercion. Departments that offer nothing of educational value in return for research participation are poor role models for budding young psychologists. Although it was difficult to assess the extent to which subject pool participants received valuable education through their participation, we did observe that subject pool policies and materials varied greatly in their emphasis on, or enforcement of, the requirement that educational value be provided to students.

Inadequate Handouts

Handouts for students and researchers who use the pools may be so densely formatted and poorly organized that they are difficult to read or comprehend. They may be devoted to "selling" students on the value of participation. They may fail to provide the details that students and researchers need to know for the research to occur in a smooth and respectful fashion.

Inadequate Administration

From the perspective of most students, the acceptability of the subject pool lies in its day-to-day handling of problems. Does a warm friendly person who possesses good judgment handle questions and problems? Students sometimes forget which study they signed up for, where it is, or at what time they are to appear. What of the students who need to know whether they have, indeed, fulfilled the entire subject pool requirement for a given course? What if a student learns at 5 p.m. that his parents, who live 3000 miles away, were in a near-fatal accident, and catches the red-eye special out of town to be with them? Is there an answering machine that will take his message that he cannot keep his subject pool appointment? Is there an efficient and compassionate procedure for excusing his failure to leave a message?

A subject pool may have an outstanding official policy, and may ensure that all subjects receive educational feedback in return for their participation, but these features pale in importance in contrast to the way the subject pool administration responds to the problems of the students who sign up to participate.

What Makes A Subject Pool Ethical?

A subject pool is probably only as ethical as the teachers, subject pool administrators, and researchers who are involved with it. It is beyond the purview of this chapter to discuss the kinds of leadership and scholarship that provide the needed intellectual and moral underpinning. Suffice it to mention that there are a number of sources of information about research ethics and relevant ethical problem solving. Two journals are devoted to relevant ethical inquiry and problem solving: *IRB: A Review of Human Research,* and *Ethics and Behavior.* The National Institutes of Health (NIH) Office for Protection From Research Risks (OPRR) collaborates with various universities and other organizations to put on workshops across the nation. Books are available that provide an in-depth foundation for ethical problem solving in social and behavioral research, including Boruch and Cecil (1979) *Assuring the Confidentiality of Social Research Data,* Renzetti and Lee (1992) *Researching Sensitive Topics,* and Sieber (1992) *Planning Ethically Responsible Research.* Faculty who have learned to integrate ethical concerns with the procedural and methodological concerns of research, and who weave this knowledge into their teaching and research practice, will have an appropriate perceptual set for developing ethical subject pool procedures. Nevertheless, subject pools are different in many ways from other research settings, and there is much that any subject pool administrator can learn from the experience of others.

There are various kinds of materials that subject pool administrators might provide to students and to researchers who use the pool. We examined all of the subject pool materials sent to us by the participants in our study. Some gave evidence of thoughtfully organized and well-managed pools, and provided a wealth of ideas. A 54-page archive document consisting of copies of exemplary documents is available from the National Auxiliary Publication Service. The main features of these exemplars are summarized, along with some specific examples, somewhat paraphrased.

Instructions to Students

The qualities that distinguished some course handouts as outstanding included a highly readable format, simplicity and clarity of rules and procedures, clarity about what is required of students who do not wish to participate in the subject pool, and respectful tone and content. The following is a brief outline of a three-page handout that Sieber and Saks (1989) found most impressive:

IMPORTANT!!! READ CAREFULLY!!!

RESEARCH REQUIREMENT: STUDENT INFORMATION SHEET

Direct All Questions to: (name, office, and office hours of person in charge)

Subject Pool Sign-Up Sheets: (location of sign-up sheets)

Psychology Subject Pool: (a paragraph on what a subject pool is)

Research Requirements: (a statement of the alternative research requirements from which students may choose)

Rights of Participants in the Subject Pool: (statement stressing conformance with APA ethical guidelines, voluntariness, confidentiality, and encouragement to ask questions about the research in which one participates)

Procedures for Subject Pool Volunteers: How do I volunteer? (sign up procedures) What if no posted study fits my schedule? What if I can't make an experiment I signed up for? What if I have questions? What if the experimenter doesn't show up?

Obtaining Credit/Deadlines for Research Requirement: How do I obtain credit for subject pool participation? How do I obtain credit for article summaries? What are the due dates?

Questions Concerning the Subject Pool and Article Summaries: To whom to direct questions. Who keeps track of your research participation? How does your research participation influence your course grade?

Some other exemplary materials distributed to students included questionnaires for students to indicate whether they were treated properly by the experimenter, announcements of the procedure for complaining, and announcements advising students on how to get the most out of research participation.

Making Participation Voluntary

Can participation in subject pools be a course requirement and still be voluntary? To comply with federal law, subject

pools have had to modify their recruitment procedures somewhat. A few make participation voluntary in the strictest
sense—anyone may volunteer with no strings attached.
More typically, however, students in one or more lower division courses have, as a course requirement, a choice among
several educational alternatives. For example, they may participate in the subject pool, attend a special lecture, watch a
movie, read and comment on some psychological literature,
experience taking some tests (e.g., personality, attitudes) and
receive an interpretation of their test results, attend a demonstration, and so forth. The educational value of each of
these choices is described to students. The alternatives are
truly valuable and nonpunitive in character. They are experiences that a good student would like to have. (An example
of a punitive alternative is being required to write a paper of
considerable length.)

Proper Treatment by the Experimenter

There are many possible approaches to discovering whether
subjects are treated respectfully and to motivating experimenters to respect those they study. Many departments have
fairly detailed statements given to anyone wishing to use the
pool, describing not just the rules of conduct required of researchers but also the philosophy or rationale underlying
those rules. In addition, departments benefit by maintaining
a bookshelf of material on research ethics including APA's
*Ethical Principles in the Conduct of Research with Human Partic-
ipants* (1992), which is currently under revision.

Given that some experimenters may regard such rules and
guidelines as bureaucratic boilerplate that can be ignored, it
is useful to ask subjects to indicate briefly in a questionnaire
whether they were treated properly. This has many advantages. It gives each student an opportunity to express how
he or she was treated. It reinforces what students should
know about the rights of human subjects, and how they,
when they become the experimenter, should treat subjects. It
provides an objective measure of how well the department
is doing with respect to treatment of subject pool partici-

pants, and indication of areas in which improvement is needed. And it indicates whether any student or faculty users of the pool are behaving unethically; this feedback can serve as grounds for warning unethical researchers or for rescinding their privilege of using the pool.

These questionnaires varied considerably in the ease with which they might be answered and reviewed, and the depth of information a student respondent might provide; as usual, ease comes at the expense of depth. The first exemplar questionnaire is easy to respond to and easy to review and tabulate, and does not call for detailed responding:

> Each participant is asked to indicate how he or she was treated after every subject pool experience by darkening the appropriate T or F circle on a scanner sheet in response to the following questionnaire. Respondents are assured anonymity.
>
> 1. The researcher was prompt and organized.
> 2. The researcher was courteous.
> 3. I was reminded at the beginning of the session that I could decline to participate in any part of the research or choose to discontinue participation at any time.
> 4. I received an explanation of the methods and purposes of the study.
> 5. In my judgment, the explanation was adequate.
> 6. The researcher either described the anticipated results of the study or told me how to obtain a description of the results at a future date.
> 7. I was informed of sources (if any) of possible stress, embarrassment, anxiety, or other discomfort beyond that which I would ordinarily expect in my day-to-day activities as a student.
> 8. I was reasonably comfortable during the study; it did not involve more anxiety, embarrassment, or other discomfort than I would ordinarily expect in my day-to-day activities as a student. If you answered FALSE to item 8, please answer item 9.
> 9. Although I felt discomfort, the researcher provided sufficient justification for the discomfort that I experienced.

If you answered FALSE to any of the above questions, would you please describe the reason(s) for your answer on the back of this sheet of paper? Also, please feel free to make any other comments you wish to convey about this study or the research participation requirement in general.

Another student questionnaire asks more of the respondent and the reviewer, and does not readily lend itself to objective scoring. Although students may use it to convey a depth of information and departments might use it as a tool for making sweeping revisions of subject pool procedures or research methods curriculum, it also invites thoughtless, uninterpretable, and nonobjective responses from the hurried or unmotivated student respondent, and invites disregard by an overburdened or unmotivated subject pool coordinator:

Please answer all of the following questions about the research project in which you just participated. Your answers are completely confidential and will not be shown to anyone. When you are finished answering all of the questions, take this slip to the Psychology Office in Room (room number).

1. Were you treated with respect and courtesy? If not, then please describe what happened.
2. Did anything about the research project disturb you? If so, then please describe what that was.
3. Did you receive both a written *and* an oral explanation of the research project?
4. Was participating in this research project a learning experience for you? Why or why not?
5. Was participating in this research project an interesting and enjoyable experience for you? Why or why not?
6. What was the major purpose or goal of this research project?

Questions and Complaints

A postexperimental questionnaire does not allow for questions or complaints that occur to the participant later. This requires a somewhat broader approach. For example, each participant might be provided with something like the following when they sign up for participation:

Getting the Most Out of Participation

A debriefing period will follow your participation in the experiment. Please feel free to ask questions during this time. You may often get as much out of the discussion following the experiment as you do during actual participation. The researchers will be more than happy to discuss any aspect of the study with you. Basically, you'll get as much out of the experience as you put into it.

By participating in this research, you are providing a very valuable service to the psychology department. Your contribution in this regard is highly valued and much appreciated. As an integral component of the research done in the psychology department, you can and should expect to be treated with respect and kindness, and to be fully debriefed at the end of the experiment. If, at any time, you are unhappy with your experience, please call me (department chair, give phone number). We would not only like to make your participation in psychological research an educational experience, but a pleasurable one as well.

Sometimes the nature of the experiment isn't fully understood, even after the experimenter or his/her assistant has attempted to explain it. If there are questions or concerns about the project that you wish to discuss at some time in the future, we ask that you contact any of these individuals in the psychology department (name of experiment director, name of assistant, chair of the psychology department, and chair of the human subjects committee).

Knowing Who Is in the Pool and Responding to the Needs of These Individuals

Respect for research participants means being responsive to their particular characteristics and interests. Two examples of populations having special characteristics are nonmajors and students with limited English proficiency.

Many nonpsychology majors take introductory psychology only because it is a requirement within their major. Their interest in psychological research may be nil; they may view the subject pool requirement as a major annoyance. The feedback or debriefing should take into account the importance of presenting to such students information that they will find useful and interesting—not the kind of technical detail that only a dedicated psychology major would welcome.

Foreign students and recent arrivals may have limited proficiency in English; their comprehension and oral communication skills are often too limited for meaningful participation in research.

What does it mean in either case to require research participation or to penalize those who do not participate? These kinds of cases underline the importance of having a range of optional interesting and educationally valuable activities from among which students may freely choose. If there is prescreening by the experimenter for special characteristics such as English language proficiency, left-handedness, musical talent, being female and over 40, being a twin, and so on, this means that some volunteers do not qualify. There should be other interesting, attractive, and convenient alternatives to fulfilling the activity requirement. Students should not feel penalized, stigmatized, or rejected.

Educational Benefit

Students participating in an experiment or other activity as part of a course requirement legitimately expect to derive something of educational value from that experience. In addition to what students may glean on their own, educational materials should be provided by the researcher. It is inappropriate to tell students to come back later and learn the findings of the experiment. Some studies are not complete until well after students have graduated. Other studies yield results that are, at best, uninteresting. In any case, a student is unlikely to remember when or where to return for results, or why it would be interesting to do so. Although it is appropriate to tell students how they may obtain the results of the study in which they participated, one should do more.

Minimally, the researcher should debrief the student by providing an engaging verbal and written description of the research. Better yet, the researcher should also provide a brief and useful summary of what is currently known about the entire topic, in terms that are understandable and useful to the student. Such a layman's version of a literature review should be written at about the level of readability and general interest of a *Reader's Digest* article.

Ideally, debriefing should be provided immediately after participation, but may have to be delayed until the experiment is completed so as not to bias future subjects.

Sound practice dictates that the subject pool administrator requires of all researchers, on application to use the subject pool, a written statement of the debriefing and educational materials they will provide to subjects.

Participants are not the only ones who can receive educational benefit through debriefing procedures. Student researchers who use the subject pool can benefit greatly by understanding the reciprocities that are appropriate to the subject–researcher relationship. A statement such as the following might be provided to users, especially student users of the subject pool:

> A student's experience as a subject can and should be a positive educational one. This does not mean that we necessarily have to design our experiments so that they are "fun" for the subjects, but rather that our experimental procedures should include a debriefing stage in which subjects are told (a) the purpose of the experiment, (b) the relation of the purpose to the conditions that they participated in, and (c) the overall results and conclusion drawn from the experiment (or where and when such information about results will be available in the future). Whenever possible, this description should be put in the standard scientific format of hypothesis, operationally defined variables, and so on. Ideally, subjects will receive this information immediately after their participation has

been terminated, but often it is not possible to give such information immediately (because of possible contamination, multiple-session experiments, and so forth). In such cases, subjects should be informed (during the experimental session) of exactly where and when such information can be obtained.

The information provided to subjects should be in plain English. Here are two versions of a debriefing, the first loaded with jargon, and the second is a "translation" of the first into plain English.

Jargon-Laden Debriefing Statement

You have just participated in a study that is concerned with a cognitive developmental task referred to as the coordination of perspectives. Jean Piaget and Barbel Inhelder developed this microspatial developmental task. It has been demonstrated to be a task that is representative of one's overall level of spatial development. This has been verified through research efforts employing cross-sectional, longitudinal, and cross-sequential designs. The study within which you have been a participant was specifically concerned with the manipulation of two independent variables: the orientation of the other observer and the dimensionality of the comparison stimuli. The dependent measures of interest included correct responses, incorrect–egocentric responses, and incorrect–correct–nonegocentric responses. It is anticipated that the findings of this study will have an impact upon the efforts of researchers concerned with macrospatial cognitive development, and environmental cognition.

Translation into English

As you know, different people may perceive the same situation differently. This creates serious problems such as interpersonal conflict, accidents, inaccurate testimony, and failure to understand and solve problems. You have just completed a task designed to measure development of the ability to view a situation from different points of

view. We manipulated where the other person stood and
we also manipulated the complexity of what you viewed.
We were interested in knowing when you were correct
as well as the way in which you were incorrect. We
wanted to know which incorrect responses were caused
by your imposing your own view on the situation. This
is part of a series of studies that we hope will lead to our
ability to help people to view situations more objectively.
We are building on what is already known about how to
increase the objectivity of perception. We have developed
a brief review of what is known about this problem already. You may have a copy of this review if you are
interested.

Creative Solutions to Typical Problems

Some kinds of psychological research pose special problems.
Two prevalent problems are use of deception and assurance
of confidentiality or anonymity. The literature on ethical
problem solving provides answers.

How does one study behavior, such as conformity, without
deception or concealment? It is not possible to study conformity behavior, placebo effects, or Hawthorne effects without deception or concealment. Yet ethics and regulations governing human research require informed consent. One
solution to this problem is to inform participants that they
cannot be told everything about the study beforehand but
will be debriefed afterward. Another is to obtain consent to
be deceived (with debriefing afterward). These and a variety
of other alternatives to deception are described in chapter 7
of Sieber (1992).

How does one ensure confidentiality or anonymity when
there are various ways in which the identity of a participant
may "leak" out? The "ballot box" technique may be used
when collecting anonymous surveys or tests. The "randomized response method" may be used when asking questions
about behavior one would not or should not acknowledge.
Boruch and Cecil (1979) provided dozens of techniques for
ensuring confidentiality or anonymity.

The creativity with which departments teach their researchers and students to solve ethical problems is testimony both to their ethical sensitivity and to their scholarship— their willingness to read and learn from the current litera- ture on ethical problem solving in social and behavioral re- search.

Procedures for All Concerned

An ethically conducted subject pool may be likened to an orchestra. The experimenters are like musicians; they need lots of guidance. Administrators of the subject pool are like conductors; they need to know how to supervise and develop the activity, bringing it to a high level of performance. It should come as no surprise, therefore, to find that exemplary subject pools have developed comprehensive procedures for experimenters, for instructors of introductory classes from which subject pool participants are drawn, for the depart- mental administrator or aide who has subject pool respon- sibilities, and for the administrator or committee of admin- istrators of the subject pool. These anonymous exemplary policies have been archived in the National Auxilary Publications Service (NAPS).[1] Drawing on these policies, I will summarize some of the policies and procedures that ex- perimenters, instructors who recruit subjects, and depart- mental administrators might emulate.

Procedures for experimenters describe the details of ethical subject pool use for which the experimenter is responsible. This includes details of gaining approval, recruitment, deal- ing with lost subjects (those who have forgotten the time or place of the experiment), instructions to subjects, giving

---

[1]This 54-page NAPS document, No. 04688, is available from NAPS c/o Microfiche Publications, P.O. Box 3513, Grand Central Station, New York, NY 10163-3513. With the order, not under separate cover, send $17.95 (U.S. funds on a U.S. bank only) for photocopies or $4.00 for microfiche. Out- side the United States and Canada, add postage of $4.50 for the first 20 pages and $1.00 for each 110 pages of material thereafter ($1.50 for mi- crofiche postage). Institutions and organizations may order by purchase order. However, there is a billing and handling charge for this service of $15.00, plus any applicable postage.

credit for participation, dealing with excused absences and "no shows" by subjects, handling experimenter no-shows, equipment breakdowns, postexperimental procedures, supervision of research assistants, and so on. Typically, to gain approval the researcher must set forth not only the details of the study, including a risk–benefit assessment, but also must present the informed consent statement, the debriefing procedure, and the precautions that are being taken to reduce risk or discomfort to participants. The recruitment procedure must be coordinated with the instructor whose class provides the subjects, and with the administrators who monitor and control the use of the subject pool.

Procedures for instructors concern their preparation for supplying subjects, their instructions to students, and their record keeping concerning student participation. Typically the instructor must provide information about the approximate number of subjects available, and about the instructors' policies regarding access to student–subjects in their classes. At the initial class meeting, the instructor makes sure students are familiar with the subject pool procedures, and distributes information describing these procedures. The instructor may allow researchers to obtain screening information from potential subjects in the classroom (e.g., demographic or personality information). The administrator of the subject pool (perhaps the departmental secretary) provides the instructor with a list of approved research projects; these are posted so that students may sign up for those in which they wish to participate. Instructors who require either subject pool participation or some other activity of each student will have certain record-keeping responsibilities, in collaboration with the subject pool administrators.

Procedures for the subject pool administrator pertain mostly to the facilitation of paperwork. The administrator must keep the needed forms on hand in adequate amounts. An estimate of the anticipated number of subjects should be obtained in advance of the term. Materials to be handed out in the first class must be prepared and given to the instructors ahead of time. The information required of experimenters must be collected and forwarded to the administrators of the subject pool for evaluation of the acceptability of their procedures. On approval, various details must be handled, such as providing sign-up sheets, credit slips (signifying participation), recording of participation, absences, no-shows, and so on, and filing of completed sign-up sheets. The administrator may maintain an answering machine to be checked daily for cancellations of subject appointments. Usually, there is a bulletin board listing approved experiments and containing sign-up sheets; this needs to be maintained, with obsolete sheets removed. The administrator serves as a general troubleshooter who detects and solves problems, referring them to the appropriate administrators as necessary.

Procedures for the subject pool administrator or committee may include evaluating use applications, allocating subject hours under conditions of high demand, or considering requests for use of the pool by investigators who are not members of the department, investigating problems, overseeing the administrator, and recommending limitation of subject pool privileges of anyone who misuses the pool.

Rather bureaucratic, isn't it?

Transforming Bureaucracy Into Education

The trick is to make these procedures meaningful. This is done through intelligent integration of ethical practice into the curriculum. The purpose of all of this is to respect the interests and well-being of participants. The process is to discover the ways in which this needs to be done. The motivation for doing so is manifold: (a) the desire to do the right thing, (b) respect or fear of sanctions for wrongdoing, (c) a sense of professionalism and responsibility, and—here's the big one—(d) an understanding that unethical practice is bad science or bad pedagogy (depending on whether one is researching or teaching). Disrespectful treatment of subjects backfires in many ways. It makes subjects lie and deceive the investigator. It produces invalid results. And it gives science a bad name.

A department steeped in ethical sensitivity and well-informed ethical problem solving is in the best position to create ethical subject pool practices. The procedures that result become meaningful, workable living documents that change and grow as dictated by changing circumstances.

Recommendations

Subject pools must be administered in compliance with federal law governing research and with the ethical code of the APA.

Instructions distributed to potential student subject pool participants should be highly readable and respectful, should outline subject pool rules and procedures in a simple and clear way, and should clearly state what is required of students who do not wish to participate in the subject pool. Alternatives to subject pool participation should be nonpunitive, educationally valuable, equitable, and attractive.

Student research participants should be asked, through a questionnaire or otherwise, whether they were treated properly. Procedures should be in place that allow student research participants to ask questions or complain at any time after the research is completed. Much of the educational benefit students derive from research participation depends on their being properly debriefed. The debriefing statement should contain, in plain English, the purpose of the experiment, the relationship of the purpose to the conditions that the students participated in, and the overall results and conclusions drawn from the experiment (or when and where such results will be available in the future). Comprehensive, meaningful procedures should be developed for experimenters, for instructors of introductory psychology classes from which subject pool participants are drawn, for the departmental secretary or other personnel who have subject pool responsibilities, and for the administrator or committee of administrators of the subject pool.

References

American Psychological Association, Committee for the Protection of Human Participants in Research. (1992). *Ethical principles in the conduct of research with human participants.* Washington, DC: Author.

Boruch, R. F., & Cecil, J. S. (1979). *Assuring confidentiality of social research data.* Philadelphia: University of Pennsylvania Press.

Kulich, R. J., Seldon, J. W., Richardson, K., & Servies, S. (1978, May). *Frequency of employing undergraduate samples in psychological research and subject reaction to forced participation.* Paper presented at the meeting of the Midwest Psychological Association, Chicago.

Renzetti, C. M., & Lee, R. (Eds.). (1992). *Researching sensitive topics.* Newbury Park, CA: Sage.

Sieber, J. E. (1992). *Planning ethically responsible research.* Newbury Park, CA: Sage.

Sieber, J. E., Iannuzzo, R., & Rodriguez, B. (1995). Deception methods in psychology: Have they changed in twenty-three years? *Ethics and Behavior, 5,* 67–85.

Sieber, J., & Saks, M. (1989). A census of subject pool characteristics and policies. *American Psychologist, 44,* 1051–1063.

II

The Research Experience From the Participant Perspective

This section provides information about ways that participants are likely to view their research experiences. Relevant issues are the benefits to students of research participation, ways in which students' research experiences can be assessed, and ways to improve student motivation to appear as agreed. These considerations are critical, not only to ensuring that participant welfare is placed foremost in importance, but also to conducting an efficient DSP.

Chapter 3 is a report of the results of a survey undertaken to indicate who participates in DSPs and why, what measurable benefits accrue to participants, how participants perceive their research experience, and how knowledgeable these participants are about DSP practices that affect them directly.

Chapter 4 details ways in which slips given to participants to demonstrate that they have participated can be used to assess their research experiences. In this regard, the types of information that can be distributed before and after research participation to enhance students' experiences are presented. Moreover, questions about participants' research experiences can be asked on the credit slips themselves, and the types of questions asked as well as representative responses are reported.

Chapter 5 answers questions about why students fail to appear as agreed to participate in research and what can be done to minimize this problem. Not only rates of nonappearance but also major reasons for nonappearance and a report of the success of measures that have been introduced to reduce nonappearance rates are reported.

In summary, this second section focuses on how it feels to be a research participant, the pros and cons of the research experience, how these can be assessed, and how to increase the reliability of participation.

Chapter

3

Research Participation Among General Psychology Students at a Metropolitan Comprehensive Public University

Bradley M. Waite and Laura L. Bowman

A prior report placed the number of psychology research articles published annually at more than 4000 (Martin, 1996). Recent online searches at our university using ULRICH's serials directory and MEDLINE estimate the number of published psychology studies using human participants to be 6700 annually (Emily Chasse, personal communications, March 26, 1996; March 21, 1997). Moreover, considering journal rejection rates and projects that are conducted but never published (e.g., student theses and projects), the number of research studies involving human participants is greater yet. Investigators have largely ignored the demands of research participation as well as the benefits. In this chapter we describe results from an ongoing empirical study of student perceptions of research (Bowman & Waite, 1997, 1998) to examine profits and liabilities that students may acquire through such involvement.

Who Participates?

Undergraduate students taking lower division courses have been the primary source of data collection for behavioral researchers. For example, Jung (1969) found that data collected from undergraduate subject pools accounted for about 90% of the total gathered at the universities he investigated. Others (Sieber & Saks, 1989) have reported that 73% to more than 90% of the articles published in selected APA journals used participants from subject pools.

Reliance on subject pools poses a threat to internal validity. In addition, questions about the demand placed on the students, the "quasi-coercive" nature of participation in some subject pools (Rosenthal, 1994), and the profits and liabilities that students face in their participation, should be answered. Research projects for which students are recruited should have been reviewed and approved (or exempted) by local Institutional Review Boards (IRB), their designate, or other locally determined review procedures (e.g., course instructors). The IRB's primary responsibility is to protect research participants by assessing the risks and benefits of proposed studies and ensuring compliance with ethical principals and federal guidelines (cf. APA, 1992; Department of Health and Human Services, 1981). In conducting risk–benefit analyses, IRBs consider potential benefits that prospective participants gain directly from the study procedures or indirectly from benefits likely to accrue to humankind. However, department subject pool policy is often predicated on the assumption that an additional class of benefit exists, namely the interest-enhancing and educational value of research participation. This study is intended to yield information relevant to this benefit type.

Research Setting

Central Connecticut State University is a metropolitan, comprehensive, public university that enrolls approximately 12,600 full- and part-time students. With the transition from college to university status in the 1980s and the concomitant evolution of the institutional mission, expectations for scholarly activity have increased. Consistent with the movement toward greater research expectation, in 1992 the Psychology

Department established its first subject pool. The goals of this department-adopted policy were to standardize and streamline research procedures and to provide "outside of classes" research experience for students that would enhance interest in psychology and have educational value.

The psychology department has 18 full-time and 14 adjunct faculty members. It has masters' programs in general and community (prevention) psychology that currently enroll approximately 30 full- and part-time students. Psychology undergraduate majors number about 500. The main subject pool users come from the ranks of faculty, graduate students, and undergraduate majors taking a second course in research methods who conduct faculty-supervised research projects. Although many of the faculty study noncollege populations, the subject pool is the primary single source for data collection.

Subject Pool Specifications

Students in general psychology are required to earn three units of research credit. Units are earned by one or any combination of three procedures: (a) participating in research projects; (b) participating in a "mass testing" session; or (c) writing brief summary and reaction papers to published research articles. In the research participation option, credit for projects varies, with one unit being earned for each half-hour (or partial half-hour) of participation. Research projects may be experimental or nonexperimental, and include a wide variety of data collection methods, with the most common tool being paper and pencil questionnaires. Each semester one or two mass testing sessions are held. During these assemblies, students respond to numerous questionnaires. They earn from two to four units of credit. During the term on which we report, one three-credit mass testing was held. Students choosing the paper option earn a maximum of two units for each article read. The paper option is roughly equivalent in terms of demand. Students are clearly informed that although the paper should be well-written, it does "not have to be a completely polished term paper" and that they should try to spend no more than an hour writing it. This relatively low time demand was created mindfully with the intent to avoid student coercion into research partici- pation while ensuring primary exposure to research and demonstrating the value placed on research by the depart- ment.

At the beginning of the semester, all general psychology students are given a handout that supplements their syllabus and describes in detail (and in summary) the research re- quirement and the presumed benefits of participation for the course. Specific detailed information about how to choose and sign-up for projects, how to submit research papers, how many units of participation are required, and how to register complaints is included. Individual instructors are asked to review the requirements with their class, which includes a discussion of their rights and the role of the IRB. Individual instructors determine how the units of credit are used and advise their students at the beginning of the semester as to their policy.

Purpose of the Study

Recently, researchers have explored the educational value of subject pools (Landrum & Chastain, 1995). However, the ed- ucational value of subject pools is difficult to quantify and assess directly (Lichtenthal, 1996). We decided to measure several components that collectively address the issue of what "profits," if any, students obtained through participa- tion in our research activities. We examined characteristics of participants in each of the research options. We assessed stu- dents' appraisals of the research dimension of the class (i.e., satisfaction). And we evaluated whether our interest- enhancement–educational goals were being met (i.e., student perceptions of psychology and research, procedural knowl- edge).

Participants

Students from 7 of the 11 sections of the general psychology course in a recent fall semester participated. A total of 210 students returned questionnaires (approximately 31% of students enrolled in general psychology that semester; 39% of the seven participating sections), of which 202 were usable for analyses. Students represented 25 different majors. The most commonly reported majors were *undecided* (n = 32), *elementary education* (n = 31) and *psychology* (n = 16); no other major exceeded n = 10. Most students attended daytime psychology classes (n = 196) and were full-time students (n = 194). A summary of participant demographic characteristics can be found in Table 3-1.

Materials

An 85-item questionnaire, divided into five sections, was employed in the assessment. Section 1 collected demographic information—age, gender, year in school, major, enrollment, and employment status. Section 2 consisted of 15 Likert-scale items that asked students their opinions about psychology (e.g., "Psychology is an important field") and research (e.g., "Research is necessary to understand human behavior"). This section also included items intended to assess students' knowledge of the specifics of the mechanisms of the subject pool, such as "I know where to go on campus to sign-up for projects if I want to participate in psychological research."

Sections 3, 4, and 5 were completed only by students who participated in the particular option being assessed. Section 3 questions focused on the research participation option, section 4 assessed the mass testing option, and section 5 assessed the paper option. Student participation in the three options was reported. Each of the three sections also included 20 items designed to assess the experiences that students accrued from participating in that particular option. For example, in section 3 students responded on a 5-point Likert scale to items designed to measure students' (a) understand-

Table 3-1

Student Participant Demography, Characteristics, and Grade Point Average

Demographic variable	N		
Gender[a]			
Women	131		
Men	69		
Class size[a]			
>90 students	114		
<90 students	86		
Employment status			
Not employed	66		
1–10 h/wk	35		
11–20 h/wk	66		
21–30 h/wk	26		
31+ h/wk	6		
Year in college			
First year	170		
Second year	19		
Third year	8		
Fourth year	3		
Fifth year +	2		
Expected grade[a]			
A, A−	46		
B+, B, B−	98		
C+, C, C−	49		
D+, D, D−	7		
F	0		
GPA	*m*	*sd*	*n*
Self-reported	2.62	0.53	138

[a]*n* may vary because of missing data from some students.

ing of the rules of research participation and their rights as research participants (e.g., "I understood that I could decline to participate in any procedure for any reason"); (b) students' perceptions of how they were treated and informed by the researcher (e.g., "The researcher was polite"); and (c) satisfaction with their experience (e.g., "Volunteering in the research projects was a rewarding experience"). Sections 4 and 5 questions were similar to those just described, except that they referred to the mass testing and paper options, respectively. Students were asked to comment (in an open-ended format) on their experiences related to the research participation, mass testing, and paper writing activities.

Procedure

Graduate assistants administered and collected the questionnaires during the final 2 weeks of a 15-week semester. All other subject pool activities had been completed by this time. Data were collected either during one in-class session or at the discretion of the instructor as a "take-home" activity that was collected at the beginning of the next class period. Procedures to ensure anonymity and confidentiality were employed. Instructors did not have access to students' responses.

Identification of Factors

Four separate principal components analyses (PCA) were performed on items in the survey to identify patterns of responding that could empirically validate the existence of underlying constructs that we believed we were measuring. That is, we wished to identify patterns reflecting perceptions of psychology, perceptions of research, satisfaction with the experience, and knowledge of procedures.

All four principal components analyses with promax rotation were performed using SAS, and in each case oblique rotation was retained because the interfactor correlations were of moderate strength. The PCAs were performed on items from sections 2 through 5 in the survey. Summary information for each PCA performed is provided in Table 3-2. In sum, we found empirical support that we were measuring

Table 3-2
Principal Components Analyses (PCA) Summary Information

PCA no.	N	Question section, no. items analyzed	Label of factors retained	No. items retained	Minimum loading
1	199	2, 15	1. Knowledge of procedures	5	(0.71)
			2. Perceptions of psychology	4	(0.71)
			3. Perceptions of research	3	(0.70)
2	145	3, 20	1. Satisfaction with research	6	(0.70)
			2. Researchers' behavior	7	(0.53)
			3. IRB rule understanding	2	(0.69)
3	76	4, 19	1. Satisfaction with mass testing	5	(0.77)
			2. Researchers' explanations	4	(0.69)
			3. Mass testing atmosphere	5	(0.69)
4	41	5, 11	1. Satisfaction with paper writing	6	(0.61)

NOTES: All retained factors had eigenvalues greater than 1. Section 2 was to be completed by all students. Sections 3, 4, and 5 were completed only by those participating in the research, mass testing, and paper options, respectively.

students' perceptions of psychology, perceptions of research, and knowledge of specific procedures concerning the research dimension, as well as students' satisfaction with the research, mass testing, and paper options.

To assess students' appraisals of the research activities and to evaluate whether our interest-enhancement–educational goals were being met, we summed individual items retained as factors from the PCA that measured the following concepts: (a) perceptions of psychology, (b) perceptions of research, (c) knowledge of specific procedures, (d) satisfaction with the research option, (e) satisfaction with the mass testing option, and (f) satisfaction with the paper-writing option. Higher scores indicate more favorable perceptions and greater satisfaction. See Table 3-2 for the number of items retained per factor.

Correlates of Research Participation

A one-way MANOVA comparing those engaged as "participants" in the research option to those who did not participate (participation status) on six dependent measures was performed. Three of the six measures were demographic variables obtained from items on the survey: employment status, class size, and expected grade. Numeric values ranging from 1 to 5 were coded for each variable. The remaining three measures were factors obtained from the PCA on section 2 reported earlier: perceptions of psychology, perceptions of research, and knowledge of specific procedures. The MANOVA indicated a significant relationship between participation status and the dependent measures (Hotelling's multivariate trace criterion ($T = 0.154$, $F\ [6, 192] = 4.92$, $p = .001$). To test each of the six measures individually, univariate ANOVAs by participation status performed on the six dependent variables (see Table 3-3) revealed significant F-values for employment status, class size, and knowledge of procedures. Perceptions of research was marginally significant ($p = .07$). Significant differences were not obtained for grade expected or percep-

Table 3-3

Means, Standard Deviations, F- and p-values of Each of the Six Dependent Measures as a Function of Participation Status

Dependent measure	Participation status		F	p
	Participated[a]	Did not participate[b]		
Employment status[*,c]	2.24 (SD = 1.11)	2.67 (SD = 1.23)	5.55	0.02
Class size[*,d]	3.03 (SD = 1.27)	2.60 (SD = 1.42)	4.27	0.04
Grade expected[e]	3.96 (SD = 0.77)	3.79 (SD = 0.80)	1.70	0.19
Perceptions of psychology[f]	16.81 (SD = 2.37)	16.31 (SD = 2.02)	1.94	0.16
Perceptions of research[g]	13.08 (SD = 1.55)	12.65 (SD = 1.38)	3.29	0.07
Knowldge of procedures[**,h]	21.86 (SD = 3.29)	19.46 (SD = 3.90)	21.29	0.00

[*]$p < .05$.
[**]$p < .001$.
[a]Total number of students who participated in research = 148; with the exception of employment status where $n = 147$.
[b]Total number of students who did not participate in research = 52.
[c]Scoring: (0 hrs = 1, 1–10 hr = 2, 11–20 hr = 3, 21–30 hr = 4, 31+ hr = 5).
[d]Scoring: (20–30 students/class = 1, 31–45 = 2, 46–90 = 3, 91–200 = 4).
[e]Scoring: (A/A− = 5; B, B+, or B− = 4; C, C+, or C− = 3; D, D+, or D− = 2; F = 1).
[f]Scoring: range = 4–20; higher numbers indicate more favorable perceptions.
[g]Scoring: range = 3–15; higher numbers indicate more favorable perceptions.
[h]Scoring: range = 5–25; higher numbers indicated greater knowledge of procedures.

tions of psychology. Effect sizes (Cohen's d) ranged from .32 to .67 for significant differences.

Results indicated that students who did participate in research: (a) were employed significantly fewer hours, (b) were enrolled in larger sections of the general psychology course, (c) had greater knowledge of the specific procedures associated with research participation, and (d) had marginally more favorable perceptions of research than those who did not participate in research.

Satisfaction Differences

We compared levels of satisfaction among those who participated in the research option, mass testing, and the paper-writing option. The PCA identified factors that measured satisfaction with each of these three experiences. However, the number and nature of the specific items that loaded on the factors made it such that direct comparison of the items was not possible. For example, the derived factor that measured satisfaction with research included six items, whereas the derived factor that measured satisfaction with mass testing included five items. To adjust for this problem, items that were common to all three factors were selected for subsequent analyses. Five items were common to all three factor structures: *had fun* (participating in research projects, mass testing, or writing), *was interesting, was rewarding, was satisfying, increased interest.* Scores were summed across these items with a range of 5 (low satisfaction) to 25 (high satisfaction).

Of the 202 total respondents, 122 reported having participated in only one of the three research options. Eighty-six students participated in a research project only, 20 participated in mass testing only, and 16 wrote a research paper only. Of the remaining 80 students, 59 took part in two of the three options, 9 reported participating in all three options, and 13 did not indicate which research options they chose. Because of the small number of students who participated in all three research options, we decided to examine the data from the 122 who reported having only one type of experience, making type of research experience a between-subjects factor. Those who indicated more than one experience type were removed from the analyses.

A one-factor between-subjects analysis of variance was performed to compare level of satisfaction among the three research options. Results indicated that differences between research participation (M = 19.12, SD = 3.80), mass testing (M = 18.05, SD = 3.38), and paper writing (M = 16.69, SD = 4.45) were marginally significant (F [2, 119] = 2.99, p = .054; η_p^2 = .05). Students who chose the paper-writing option were least satisfied with their experience.

Narrative Comments

A total of 64 students wrote at least one narrative comment about their experiences while participating in the research activities. There were a total of 46 comments about research participation, 17 comments about mass testing participation, 17 comments about writing research papers, and one comment was vague in reference (and thus removed from subsequent analyses), yielding 80 separate usable comments.

An independent observer was recruited to code the responses as being either positive (*favorable*) or negative (*unfavorable*) in nature. The observer classified comments based on the overall impression the respondent was judged to have had. One of the authors also independently coded the responses as being positive or negative using the same criterion. Interrater reliability was 98.75%

Results indicated an overwhelming number of favorable responses regarding the research participation option. There were 39 positive comments and 7 negative comments about participating as a volunteer. A chi-square test revealed significant differences in frequency of positive and negative responses (χ^2[1, N = 46] = 22.26, p < .001). The majority of positive comments described how enjoyable or rewarding the experience was (e.g., "I enjoyed volunteering in the research projects. They were well put together and the researchers always knew exactly what they were doing and were very polite. I think that participating in them has increased my interest in the field of Psych and would like to see even more projects done"). There were 11 positive comments and 6 negative comments about participating in mass testing, and 11 positive comments and 6 negative comments about writing the research paper. Chi-square tests revealed no significant differences in the frequency of response types in either condition ($\chi^2[1, N = 17] = 1.47, p > .10$).

Conclusion

The purpose of this study was to measure general psychology students' perceptions of psychology and research, their knowledge of specifics relating to the subject pool, satisfaction with research activities, and individual characteristics that might be associated with participation in our research activities. We found significant relationships between participation status and employment status, class size, and knowledge of procedures; marginal differences for perceptions of research; and no significant differences for grade expected and perceptions of psychology.

Those who did not participate in research were employed significantly more hours than those who did participate in research. This suggests that we must maintain our other research options that may be more accessible to students who work more hours and may not be available during the daytime when most of the research projects are conducted. We may need to encourage researchers to conduct their projects at a wider variety of times.

Those who participated in research were enrolled in larger sections of the general psychology course. Individual differences among professors in the way the research options were presented could account for this outcome. Instructors who teach courses that have a research participation component should be familiar with the need for and value of human research, as well as the specific mechanics associated with the process—for example, where to go to sign up to be a volunteer. Furthermore, presentation of the research options should be standardized across sections.

Those who participated in research had greater knowledge of the specific procedures associated with research participation. Thus those who served as volunteers were more confident in their knowledge of where to go to sign up for projects and deliver papers, the number of units they needed to earn, and were more likely to indicate that the research option was fully explained and that the handout explaining the procedures was clear. This may mean that a thorough understanding of the procedures may lead to greater participation, although we cannot firmly determine the directionality of this relationship.

Those who participated in research had marginally more favorable perceptions of research than those who did not participate in research ($p = .07$). Those who participated in research had slightly stronger endorsement of the ideas that research is necessary to understand human behavior, psychologists need to do research to understand why people behave in certain ways, and researchers rely on volunteers to participate in their experiments. Given that the means of both groups were quite high (refer to Table 3-3), we can conclude that students had favorable perceptions of research regardless of having participated as a volunteer.

Expected grade did not differ between those who participated in research and those who did not, suggesting no direct link between participation and learning. Of course, those who did not choose the research participation option could have decided to write a paper or participate in mass testing to bolster their grades. It is also possible that students learned concepts that did not translate easily into increased examination performance. Perceptions of psychology did not differ between those who participated and those who did not. Scores were high (see Table 3-3), indicating that students agreed that *psychology is an important field, everyone should take a course in psychology, psychology is an interesting topic*, and *learning about psychology is exciting*. It is possible that students who enroll in psychology courses already hold these opinions, or that students develop these opinions throughout the semester. Nevertheless, participation in research does not appear to have an influence on endorsement of these ideas.

Satisfaction score differences between those who participated in research, mass testing, and paper writing were marginally significant ($p = .054$) indicating that those who participated in research were more satisfied than those who wrote a paper. This, taken together with the narrative comments about participating in research (which contained significantly more positive than negative comments), leads us to believe that our students perceived this opportunity as a valuable contribution to their interest in and understanding of psychology as well as simply being fun and rewarding. Given that the satisfaction scores for all three research options were high, we believe that the experiences, particularly the research volunteer option, are positive.

Examination of the interfactor correlation between *satisfaction with research* and *researcher's behavior* reveals a moderate positive relationship ($r = 0.31$) among those who volunteered in the research. Furthermore, among those who participated in mass testing, *satisfaction with mass testing option* was moderately correlated ($r = 0.33$) with *researcher's explanations* and with *mass testing atmosphere* ($r = 0.34$), indicating that, consistent with Britton (1979), thorough and polite researchers can contribute greatly to a positive research experience.

The outcome of this study implies that there are important demographic characteristics that may influence participation in research and when evaluating or considering implementation of a subject pool, the relevance of these characteristics at one's home institution should be weighed. For instance, the relationship between participation and student employment is more problematic in academic settings where many students have external employment.

Future research should include the assessment of perceptions and knowledge both before and after student participation in research activities, and compare outcomes to students who did not participate in any research options. This would provide a more controlled assessment of the impact of the research options on students' experiences. The generalizability of our findings should also be explored.

In sum, we identified factors that empirically measured students' perceptions of psychology, perceptions of research, knowledge of specific procedures concerning the research dimension, and satisfaction with each of the three research options. We found that although students who participated in the subject pool did not perform better academically, they were generally satisfied with their experiences and found them to be rewarding. This outcome runs counter to the concern espoused by some that participation in subject pools is damaging or not useful.

Based on our results and experience we make the following recommendations to departments looking to create or revise subject pool procedures and policies:

- Retain subject pools. They appear to provide a valuable function for participants and researchers.
- Have a variety of equally attractive research options and alternatives scheduled at a variety of times.
- Make the instructions and explanations of specific procedures associated with research options clear and easy to understand (e.g., where to go to sign up to participate, how to turn in papers, how credit is assigned).
- Standardize the instructions and explanations of specific procedures associated with research options across sections.
- Direct researchers to thoroughly explain the background and purpose of their studies to contribute to the learning experience and satisfaction of participants.
- Encourage researchers to thoroughly explain any contributions to science and society that students are making by participating.
- Instruct researchers to be polite, courteous, and professional.

References

American Psychological Association. (1992). *Ethical principles in the conduct of research with human participants.* Washington, DC: Author.

Bowman, L., & Waite, B. M. (1997, May). *Is student research participation related to knowledge and perceptions of psychology and research?* Poster presented at the Midwestern Psychological Association meeting, Chicago.

Bowman, L., & Waite, B. M. (1998). [A time-lag study of student satisfaction with research activities]. Unpublished raw data.

Britton, B. K. (1979). Ethical and educational aspects of participating as a subject in psychology experiments. *Teaching of Psychology, 6,* 95–98.

Department of Health and Human Services. (1981). Final regulations amending basic HHS policy for the protection of human research subjects. *Federal Register, 46,* 8366–8391.

Jung, J. (1969). Current practices and problems in the use of college students for psychological research. *The Canadian Psychologist, 9,* 59–66.

Landrum, R. E., & Chastain, G. (1995). Experiment spot checks: A method for assessing the educational value of undergraduate participation in research. *IRB: A Review of Human Subjects Research, 17,* 4–6.

Lichtenthal, P. (1996, June 17). Undergraduate research pools. *Educational materials for: Ethical and Regulatory Issues in Social and Behavioral Science and Health Services Research, PRIM&R Proceedings, 54–57.*

Martin, D. W. (1996). *Doing psychology experiments* (4th ed). Pacific Grove, CA: Brooks/Cole.

Rosenthal, R. (1994). Science and ethics in conducting, analyzing, and reporting psychological research. *Psychological Science, 5,* 127–134.

Sieber, J. E., & Saks, M. J. (1989). A census of subject pool characteristics and policies. *American Psychologist, 44,* 1053–1061.

Evaluating Students' Research Experiences Via Credit Slips

Richard L. Moreland

As has been noted in previous chapters, most psychology departments require the undergraduate students in their introductory courses to participate in research projects (Diamond & Reidpath, 1992; Lindsay & Holden, 1987; Sieber & Saks, 1989). Although such requirements may seem simple, they can create a variety of problems for students, instructors, and researchers. To minimize those problems, many departments develop complex administrative systems, known colloquially as "subject pools." Every subject pool is unique, reflecting the ways in which a particular department tries to cope with its problems. One problem faced by nearly all subject pools is keeping track of which students have participated in which research projects. Credit slips, which are written receipts given to students for proof of participation, often provide the solution. The purpose of this chapter is to describe a special feature of the subject pool in my department—namely the use of credit slips as a tool for evaluating students' research experiences. To put that practice in con-

This is a good opportunity to thank Jim Kerrigan, and especially Kathy Freund, for their valuable assistance with subject pool operations in my department.

text, I will begin by describing the general operation of the subject pool at the University of Pittsburgh. Then I will describe the way our credit slips are designed to provide feedback about students' research experiences, and I will summarize some of the information we have gathered about these experiences. Finally, I will describe some advantages of using credit slips in this way.

Operating a Subject Pool

My department encourages students to participate in research projects for two reasons. First, research participation has educational value, especially for students who are just beginning to study psychology. Through participating in a project, listening to a researcher explain the purpose of that project, and asking questions about their research experience, students can gain valuable insights into such issues as how variables are operationalized, what factors affect the internal and external validity of research, how data are analyzed to test hypotheses, and so on. Students can also learn about specific psychological phenomena. Some of these may be unfamiliar to students, and even prosaic phenomena can seem new and exciting when students learn (through debriefing) about relevant theory and research. Finally, research participation allows students to discover what kinds of research the psychologists at their own university are conducting. Such knowledge can be useful for students who later decide to major in psychology, and perhaps make it a career. A second reason to require research participation from students, of course, is that it enables faculty and graduate students in departments such as mine to do far more research than would otherwise be possible. As a science, psychology cannot progress without such research. Some fortunate researchers have grant funds that allow them to pay people for participating in their projects, whereas other researchers somehow persuade people to volunteer as participants. But neither of these practices can generate enough participants for all the projects that researchers want to conduct. My department thus requires students to participate in research projects, viewing the students as collaborators in an important process that benefits everyone involved, and perhaps others as well.

For many years now, I have served as director of my department's subject pool. There are actually three pools each year, reflecting the semesters (fall, spring, summer) when introductory psychology courses are taught. Although the subject pool changes somewhat from one semester to another, let me offer a prototypical description of its operation. First, several weeks before a semester begins, I learn how many introductory psychology courses will be taught, and how many students are likely to be enrolled in those courses. Then I contact all of the course instructors, reminding them about the requirement for research participation (every section of introductory psychology has this requirement), and providing them with materials (to be described shortly) for their students about the requirement. Introductory psychology is taught in both daytime and evening courses, which differ in several ways. Nevertheless, we require *all* of the students enrolled in these courses to participate in 5 hours of research each. (Optional assignments, which I will describe later, are available for students who prefer not to become research participants.) Multiplying the total number of such students by five thus produces an estimate of how many hours are available for distribution to researchers.

At about the same time, several weeks before the semester begins, I send subject pool application packets to all the faculty and graduate students (about 150 people) in my department. To submit an application, a researcher must first fill out a form that provides me with information about how many students and student hours are needed for the proposed project, what kinds of students can participate, where the project is located, and who to contact if problems arise. Graduate students must also name a faculty sponsor and note whether the proposed project is meant to satisfy a degree requirement. Any grant funding for the project must also be noted, and if a project is funded, then evidence of Institutional Review Board approval must be provided.

With this form, each applicant also submits (a) a brief description of his or her research procedures, (b) a feedback sheet, and (c) a sign-up folder. A brief description of research procedures is necessary because, under the auspices of my university's Institutional Review Board, I evaluate unfunded research projects for possible risks to participants. Few of these projects involve more than minimal risks, and when they do, I can often persuade the researchers to make procedural changes that will solve the problem. Otherwise, I ask the Institutional Review Board for its evaluation of such projects. A feedback sheet is a written explanation of a research project that is given (along with a brief oral explanation) to every student during the debriefing period that follows every research session. A good feedback sheet, in my opinion, makes it clear why the project was important, what hypotheses were tested, and how a student's experiences produced data relevant to those hypotheses. Feedback sheets should also provide at least one reference to an accessible paper on the phenomenon being studied, and contact information for students who may want to discuss a project further with its director. In my experience, feedback sheets often require some revision, but researchers are usually willing to make the necessary changes, perhaps because they also want to make research participation educational for students. Finally, a sign-up folder is simply a manila file folder that provides advance information about a research project for students who might want to participate in it. The front cover of the folder contains a code number, along with information about the project's director (name and phone number), and its location, restrictions, and credit value (1 to 5 hours). Inside the folder is a brief description of the project, and some system by which interested students can make appointments for research sessions.

When a subject pool application is approved, I send the researcher a letter noting the project's code number, summarizing how many students and hours were allotted to that project, and reviewing a few general procedural guidelines. The researcher also receives an appropriate number of credit slips, and some no-show slips that can be used to penalize any students who fail to keep their appointments. Researchers are asked to post their sign-up folders on a public bulletin board, outside the department's undergraduate advising office, where students from the introductory psychology courses can review their options and make choices about the projects in which they want to participate.

In the fall and spring, 40 to 50 research projects are typically approved. These vary widely, but the modal project is a 1-hour laboratory experiment in cognitive or social psychology. Individual project allotments can range from 20 to 750 student hours. I often overbook the subject pool by about 10%, because some research projects never materialize, and other projects are never completed. A related problem is the perennial imbalance between the supply of students and the demand for them. Sometimes there are too few projects, given the total number of students enrolled in introductory psychology courses. At other times there are too many projects. Rather than changing the research participation requirement from one semester to the next, I try to solve these problems in other ways. When there are too few projects, for example, I encourage researchers from my department to propose new projects, or to accept more students for projects that were already approved. I may also contact people from other departments, if they seem to be doing (or have done) interesting research with a psychological flavor, and invite them to submit project proposals. Different tactics are needed when there are too many research projects. When that problem arises, I rely on a priority scheme that favors graduate students working on projects meant to satisfy requirements. These projects are given full allotments of student hours. Whatever subject pool resources remain are divided evenly among the other projects, with an upper limit on the total allotment that any one researcher can receive.

Approval letters and materials are sent to researchers by the end of the first week of the semester. At about the same time, instructors of the introductory psychology courses are asked to distribute and discuss with their students the subject pool materials that I referred to earlier. These materials include handouts describing the research participation requirement, and flyers describing optional assignments for students who prefer not to participate in research projects.

The handouts begin by explaining why my department requires students to participate in research projects. The requirement itself is then described, along with the consequences of noncompliance. Students are told that if they earn a passing grade in introductory psychology, but do not satisfy the requirement by the end of the semester, then they will be given an incomplete grade that remains on their transcript until the requirement has been satisfied. (Students who fail the course simply receive an "F" grade, whether they satisfy the requirement or not.) Next, the handout instructs students on how to arrange to participate in research projects, namely by visiting the advising office, reviewing whatever sign-up folders are posted there, and making appointments for sessions in the projects that seem most interesting. The handout then summarizes the benefits and risks of participating in research projects, and students' privileges and responsibilities as research participants. Research participation is described as enjoyable and educational, with few or no risks, other than the possibility of deception in some projects. An important privilege is the ability to quit a research project at any time, and for any reason, without loss of credit or other penalties. Students are also promised a full debriefing, both oral and written, at the end of every research session. An important responsibility is to keep appointments and to arrive for them on time. When students want to cancel an appointment, or expect to be more than 10 minutes late, they must contact the researcher or call a special subject pool hotline at least an hour in advance. Otherwise, they can be penalized for the number of credit hours they would have earned. The handout then goes on to explain how credit slips are used for recording and evaluating students' research participation, and mentions optional paper assignments (described in the flyers) for students who would rather satisfy the requirement in other ways. A deadline, usually the end of the semester, is then named, by which all credit slips and papers must be submitted for review. The handout closes with an invitation for students who have research participation problems to contact me, either directly or through the subject pool hotline.

The flyers describe an optional assignment that is available to all students. Briefly, we ask them to write a paper summarizing a magazine or newspaper article about psychology. The paper, which must be typewritten (double-spaced) and at least 300 words long, should review the contents of that article and then relate it to issues covered in the introductory psychology course. Writing such a paper takes about an hour for most students, so each paper that is submitted earns a student one credit hour. The entire research participation requirement can be satisfied in this way, or students can combine writing papers with participating in research projects.

As the semester progresses, levels of research participation rise and fall. Some students attempt to satisfy their requirement immediately, but most of them wait until the very end of the semester. Few students sign up for appointments around vacation periods or during midterm examinations. I try to review the sign-up folders on a regular basis, to ensure there are enough research projects available for the students, and to get some sense of how many students are participating (and which projects they seem to prefer). It is often necessary for me to remind the researchers and the students about their obligations—it sometimes seems that if researchers are not complaining about how few students are signing up for their projects, then the students are complaining about how few research projects are available to them. Toward the end of the semester, I provide the introductory psychology instructors with weekly reports summarizing the progress each of their students has made toward satisfying the research participation requirement. They are asked to make these reports accessible to students, so that problems can be identified before the semester ends. A final report is later issued to each instructor, so that course grades (reflecting students' compliance with the requirement) can be prepared for the university registrar. At about this time, a general report on the subject pool's operation is also sent to all researchers and instructors.

Table 4-1 illustrates the success of my department's subject pool. The table summarizes subject pool operations since 1990; few students take introductory psychology in the summer, so only data for fall and spring semesters are shown. Several aspects of the table are worth noting. First, the compliance rate among students is fairly high, averaging about

Table 4-1

Subject Pool Operations

School year and term	Number of students	Compliance (percentage)	Papers (percentage)	Penalties (percentage)
1990, 1	1650	87	3	7
1990, 2	1000	81	4	12
1991, 1	1750	82	6	16
1991, 2	850	82	6	13
1992, 1	1250	84	4	18
1992, 2	900	80	5	14
1993, 1	1260	80	3	9
1993, 2	850	85	2	8
1994, 1	1275	79	14	15
1994, 2	880	80	10	13
1995, 1	1320	78	9	17
1995, 2	875	83	11	17
1996, 1	1500	78	7	27
1996, 2	830	76	13	14
1997, 1	1650	75	17	15
1997, 2	825	77	14	15
1998, 1	1800	78	19	11
1998, 2	850	79	69	12

NOTE: 1990, 1 and 1990, 2 refer (respectively) to the fall and spring semesters of the 1989–90 school year; the other dates should be interpreted accordingly. The remaining columns show the total number of students participating in each pool, the proportion of students who completed the requirement, and the proportions of students who wrote at least one optional paper or were penalized at least once.

80%. I have, once or twice, investigated noncompliance and found that about half of the students who failed to satisfy their research participation requirement also failed their introductory psychology courses. So the "true" rate of compliance is probably more than 90%. About half of the students who receive incomplete course grades because of noncompliance try to satisfy the requirement quickly, within just a week or two after the semester ends. The remaining students work at a far more leisurely pace, sometimes sending me the necessary credit slips or papers much later. Within a period of about 3 years, nearly everyone who received an incomplete grade satisfies the requirement and finally gets the course grade that was actually earned. Another noteworthy aspect of the table is the proportion of students who wrote one or more papers, rather than participating in research projects. This proportion is rather low, averaging about 9%, but fluctuates considerably over time. A final aspect of the table worth noting is the proportion of students who are penalized at least once for such misbehavior as arriving late for research sessions or skipping them altogether. This proportion is also low, averaging about 14%, and also fluctuates considerably over time.

These data suggest that our subject pool is successful, in the sense that most students do satisfy the research participation requirement without much trouble. But other criteria should be considered too, especially the educational value of students' research experiences. To explore that issue, let me now describe my department's use of credit slips as a tool for evaluating those experiences.

Better Uses for Credit Slips

Every subject pool must somehow cope with the problem of keeping accurate records of students' research participation. This problem can be solved in several ways, including the practice of providing students with credit slips for each of the research projects in which they participate. These slips serve as receipts that students can submit to the department as proof that they have satisfied their research participation requirement, or hold in reserve (if research participation records are kept in other ways) in case disagreements arise about how much work has actually been done. In my department, however, credit slips are used in an innovative and more productive way.

A sample credit slip from the subject pool is shown in Figure 4-1. Students receive one of these slips after every research project in which they participate. They are asked to take such slips home, answer the questions about their research experiences, and then bring the completed slips to the department's advising office. Students who fail to answer any of the questions on a credit slip receive no credit for the relevant project. They are recontacted by me and asked to complete the slip more carefully. The contents of all credit slips are completely confidential. In particular, researchers never see these slips again after distributing them to the students who participate in their projects.

As the credit slips arrive in the advising office, they are processed and entered into a computerized database (Microsoft Excel). Processing involves coding students' answers to the first five questions on the credit slips as a series of ones (*yes*) and zeros (*no*).[1]

Many students write little more than yes or no in answering these questions anyway, but some students are more loquacious. We read these more complex answers carefully, but still code them in this simple way—the workload of processing thousands of credit slips makes it impractical to do much more. Coding students' answers to the final question on the credit slips is a bit more difficult. A score of zero is given to answers implying a poor understanding of a research project. Such answers include nonanswers (blanks), claims of ignorance, vague statements or misstatements, and

---

[1]We have not checked the reliability with which students' answers to the credit slips questions are coded. However, the people who do that coding have no special interest in the results, either at a general level (in terms of the subject pool as a whole) or at the level of specific research projects.

Name: _____ Date: _____

Student ID #: _____ Instructor: _____

Project Code: _____ Project Director: _____

Credit Hours: _____

Please answer all of the following questions about the research project in which you just participated. Your answers are completely confidential and will not be shown to anyone. When you have completed this slip, take it to the Psychology Advising Office and turn it in.

- Were you treated with courtesy and respect? If not, then what happened?

- Did anything about the project disturb you? If so, then what was it?

- Did you receive both written and oral explanations of the project?

- Was participating in this project a learning experience? Why or why not?

- Was participating in this project an enjoyable experience? Why or why not?

- What was the purpose of this project?

Figure 4-1. A sample subject pool credit slip. A researcher fills in the project's code number, the name of the project's director, and the number of credit hours earned by the student. The remaining information is supplied by the student, who also answers the open-ended questions on the slip.

attempts at humor. Answers implying fair understanding of a research project are given a score of one. Such answers specify both the independent and dependent variables in a project, as well as its hypothesis. Finally, a score of two is given to answers implying a good understanding of a research project. Such answers are more detailed, often including comments about why the project was conducted, how different patterns of results would be interpreted, what the project's strengths and weaknesses seem to be, and so on. Of course, processing credit slips also involves recording each student's name, social security number, and instructor, along with the code numbers and credit hours for the relevant projects. The database contains other information as well, including penalties imposed on students by researchers (using the no-show slips), and corresponding requests by some students to have such penalties removed.

The first three questions on the credit slips focus on how students were treated by researchers. A summary of the students' answers to these questions (since 1990) can be found in Table 4-2. The data suggest that we have few problems in this regard. For example, nearly all the students say that they are treated well: The average proportion of yes answers to the first credit slip question is about 99%. In fact, many of the table entries for this question could have been rounded to 100%, but I thought that would be misleading, because there are always *some* complaints about poor treatment. I make every effort to contact the students who make such complaints and inquire about their experiences, taking action (e.g., apologizing to the student, discussing the problem with the researcher) whenever that seems warranted.

And students are seldom disturbed by their research experiences: The average proportion of yes answers to the second credit slip question is only about 6%. Student complaints in this instance usually involve minor problems, such as physical discomfort (research rooms that are too hot or cold, too bright or dim), boredom (tasks that are too dull), or workload (tasks that take too much time or energy). But sometimes the problems are more troubling, such as a researcher who acts rudely or who pressures students to do something

Table 4-2

Students' Reactions to Research Projects

School year and term	Treated well?	Problems? (percentage)	Feedback? (percentage)	Enjoyable? (percentage)	Educational (percentage)
1990, 1	99	6	91	76	77
1990, 2	99	7	99	74	72
1991, 1	99	7	98	74	78
1991, 2	98	5	96	70	74
1992, 1	99	5	97	77	78
1992, 2	99	6	98	79	79
1993, 1	99	7	98	77	78
1993, 2	99	6	99	79	80
1994, 1	97	6	97	69	72
1994, 2	99	6	98	72	70
1995, 1	99	4	96	74	78
1995, 2	99	5	96	75	79
1996, 1	99	6	97	70	76
1996, 2	99	7	98	71	75
1997, 1	99	7	94	70	76
1997, 2	99	5	98	72	74
1998, 1	97	7	94	65	68
1998, 2	95	4	93	65	65

NOTES: Entries show the proportions of students who answered "yes" to each of the first five questions on the credit slips. The unit of analysis is the credit slip rather than the student. Note that the number of students associated with each row of these tables is unclear, because students can submit different numbers of credit slips, depending on their individual patterns of research participation. One student, for example, might submit a single credit slip for a research project worth 5 credit hours. Another student might submit three slips, two for projects worth one hour apiece, and the third for a project worth 3 hours. Some students, such as those who must work off penalties, submit credit slips worth more than 5 hours in total. Capturing these complexities statistically would be difficult, but it probably is not necessary for the present purposes, which are descriptive rather than inferential.

they would rather not do. Once again, I investigate such matters carefully and take appropriate action when necessary.

Finally, the students nearly always receive both written and oral feedback about the research projects in which they participate, as subject pool policies require. The average proportion of yes answers to this third credit slip question is about 96%. Special circumstances cause at least some of the feedback problems that students experience. For example, students are occasionally dismissed from a research project early because of equipment failures, or because researchers have overbooked them to ensure groups of a certain size. In these situations, students are given credit slips, but they may not receive much feedback, because they did not actually participate.

The fourth and fifth questions on the credit slips focus on the quality of students' research experiences. The data suggest that the department has few problems in this regard either. The average proportion of yes answers to these questions is about 73% and 75%, respectively. If a project seems unenjoyable or uneducational to many students, then I work with the researcher to make suitable changes. It is difficult to make projects more enjoyable, although some researchers are willing to try. But many projects can be made more educational, if researchers develop better oral and written debriefing procedures.

On the whole, the data in Table 4-2 are encouraging. If the students' answers to the credit slip questions can be taken at face value, then there is little evidence that research participation is harmful, and some evidence that it is beneficial. Another interesting aspect of these data is their stability over time. Despite considerable turnover among both students and researchers since 1990, answers to the credit slip questions remain about the same from one semester to the next. This could be interpreted in several ways, but I believe that it reflects the influence of an administrative system that works well, and has itself remained fairly stable over time.

Clearer evidence for the educational value of student research participation in my department can be found in Table 4-3, which summarizes students' answers to the final ques-

Table 4-3

Students' Understanding of Research Projects

School year and term	Level of understanding		
	Poor	Fair	Good
1990, 1	29	66	5
1990, 2	26	67	7
1991, 1	23	70	7
1991, 2	27	61	12
1992, 1	15	78	7
1992, 2	11	76	13
1993, 1	7	86	7
1993, 2	9	81	10
1994, 1	11	83	6
1994, 2	8	86	6
1995, 1	7	89	4
1995, 2	6	90	4
1996, 1	3	92	5
1996, 2	2	91	7
1997, 1	2	88	10
1997, 2	4	86	10
1998, 1	4	91	5
1998, 2	3	94	3

NOTES: Answers to the last question on the credit slips were evaluated using the criteria described in the text. Entries show the percentages of students whose understanding of the purposes for their research participation seemed to be *poor, fair,* or *good.* The unit of analysis is the credit slip rather than the student. Note that the number of students associated with each row of these tables is unclear, because students can submit different numbers of credit slips, depending on their individual patterns of research participation. One student, for example, might submit a single credit slip for a research project worth 5 credit hours. Another student might submit three slips, two for projects worth one hour apiece, and the third for a project worth 3 hours. Some students, such as those who must work off penalties, submit credit slips worth more than 5 hours in total. Capturing these complexities statistically would be difficult, but it probably is not necessary for the present purposes, which are descriptive rather than inferential.

tion on the credit slips. On the average, students have a poor understanding of about 12% of the research projects in which they participate, a fair understanding of about 82% of those projects, and a good understanding of about 6% of the projects. These data are again encouraging—students seem to learn something from their research experiences nearly 90% of the time. And here there has been some change over the years, with a steady decline in how often students reveal a poor understanding of the projects in which they participate. This healthy change can be attributed to dedicated efforts by all of the researchers in my department to improve their debriefing procedures.

Is This Practice Worthwhile?

Before I urge other psychology departments to use credit slips in this way, let me review some of the advantages and disadvantages that ought to be considered. A major disadvantage is that using credit slips to evaluate students' research experiences requires considerable time and energy. When a thousand or so students submit several credit slips apiece, the task of processing all those data can be daunting. Many hours of work are required, and that work must be done carefully, because important outcomes for many people (students, instructors, researchers) depend on the resulting database. The task is made even more challenging by students who procrastinate, postponing research participation until late in the semester or who participate earlier in the semester but hang onto their credit slips until the semester ends. Sometimes we receive nearly half of all the credit slips during the very last week of a semester. These slips must be processed quickly, so that a final research participation report can be prepared and sent to the introductory psychology instructors. The credit slips could be computerized using optical scanning forms, of course, or we could just sample the students' research experiences, rather than trying to evaluate them all, but these labor-saving alternatives would yield weaker evidence about issues that we view as important.

There are several advantages to using credit slips for evaluating students' research experiences. The most important of these may be learning how research participation actually affects students. It is very easy to speculate about such effects, or to rely on hearsay from a few students or researchers. Credit slips can provide much better evidence about what is really going on. That evidence may not always be pleasant—credit slips occasionally reveal serious problems. But once those problems have been identified, attempts can be made to solve them, and if those attempts succeed, everyone benefits. In my opinion, any psychology department that requires students to participate in research projects should make some effort to collect data on their experiences. Such data can be collected in several ways, but credit slips are an effective option.

Another advantage of this practice is detecting problems with students or research projects more rapidly, in time to prevent any problems from becoming more serious. For example, I sometimes see credit slips early in the semester from students who simply hate the idea of participating in research projects. They describe themselves as "guinea pigs," argue that the requirement has no educational value and serves only to further the research careers of the faculty, and even threaten legal action to force changes in department policy. I often try to contact these students and gently persuade them that research participation is not so awful. I suggest that the relationship between most researchers and students is really collaborative, rather than exploitative; that students often describe their research experiences as enjoyable and educational; and that requiring research participation from students is no worse than the requirements (e.g., laboratory work, field observations) associated with other science courses at the university. My persuasion attempts are not always successful, but they succeed often enough to make them seem worthwhile. Credit slips submitted early in the semester can also reveal problems involving particular research projects. For example, the tasks that students perform in some project may prove unexpectedly stressful for them, or the researcher may behave in ways that seem to intimidate students. Problems such as these lead me to contact researchers and persuade them to change their procedures in suitable ways. Most researchers are cooperative in this regard. In fact, they are often surprised to discover that such problems exist. Few students complain about a project while it is in progress (Orne, 1962), so without the information provided by the credit slips, some research participation problems might never be detected.

Unless they collaborate on projects, researchers in most psychology departments are only vaguely aware of one another's research practices. Some researchers have better reputations than others, but the criteria for making such distinctions are often unclear. Yet another advantage of using credit slips to evaluate students' research experiences is developing normative standards for everyone involved in the subject pool. As I noted earlier, all of the researchers and instructors in the department receive a general report on subject pool operations at the end of each semester. This report contains extensive information about every research project and introductory psychology course. For example, answers to the credit slip questions by students who participated in each project are reviewed, as are the rates at which students from each course satisfied the research participation requirement, wrote papers for that purpose, and were penalized for misbehavior.

This information is helpful in at least two ways. First, it encourages informal social comparisons (Wood, 1989) among researchers and instructors, comparisons that may lead people whose performance is relatively poor to improve their practices. Second, I begin each new semester by studying the old semester's subject pool report and identifying any researchers or instructors whose performance seems problematic. I then meet with these persons to discuss those problems and offer some suggestions for improvement. If a researcher is uncooperative, then his or her access to the subject pool can be restricted. Fortunately, action of that sort has never been necessary.

Because the students' research experiences are evaluated every semester, it is also possible to look for trends in those experiences and to assess the impact of proposed changes in subject pool policies. This advantage became apparent in 1994, when a proposal was made to increase the requirement for research participation from 4 to 5 hours. There was much discussion of this proposal, and most of the arguments were very speculative. We decided to go ahead and increase the requirement for a trial period of 1 year, and then analyze whether and how that change altered the students' research experiences. As the tables suggest, no harm was done. The proportion of students who satisfied the research participation requirement declined a bit, and writing papers became somewhat more popular, but there was no clear change in penalty rates or in the kinds of research participation problems that the credit slips measure. Students were less likely to describe their research experiences as enjoyable, but descriptions of how educational those experiences were did not appear to change, and students' understanding of the research projects actually improved. All of this persuaded us to retain the new research participation requirement.

A similar situation arose in 1997, when one of the introductory psychology instructors proposed that we reduce the research participation requirement from 5 to 3 hours. He argued that requiring first- and second-year students to do so much "extra" work was burdensome and might foster negative attitudes toward psychology. This proposal was rejected, but when that instructor hinted that he might remove his students from the subject pool altogether, a compromise was soon reached by reducing the requirement to 4 hours. The effects of this change were more complex, although it is too early to be certain what is happening. As the tables show, the proportion of students who satisfied the research participation requirement did improve, and penalty rated declined. But there were also disturbing changes, especially in 1997–98 in (a) students' beliefs that they were treated well by researchers, (b) how often students reported receiving feedback about research projects, and (c) how enjoyable and educational research participation seemed to students. Students' understanding of the research projects, however, continued to improve. We will continue to monitor these changes carefully and investigate them more carefully if necessary.

Finally, the research participation requirement in my department has been challenged occasionally by students, parents, and administrators. These challenges usually focus on the educational value of participating in research projects. Evidence about that issue, obtained from the credit slips, has been useful for countering these challenges. The mere fact that we collect and analyze such data suggests a real concern for the students' welfare. And, of course, the data themselves reveal that few students have trouble satisfying the requirement, that problems arising from research participation are rare, and that for many students, participating in research projects is indeed educational, even enjoyable. Faced with such evidence, critics of the requirement have often changed their minds and acknowledged that research participation may well have some benefits for students from introductory psychology courses.

A surprising challenge to the subject pool occurred in 1997, when one member of our faculty (the same person who proposed reducing the research participation requirement to 3 hours) argued that students should not be required to participate in research at all. He proposed instead to make research participation an extra credit option. After considerable discussion, the decision was made to investigate this issue by performing an experiment. The students in this instructor's fall class were required to participate in research (4 hours per person), whereas the students in his spring class were simply encouraged to take part in research (no optional papers were permitted) as a way of earning extra credit. Several outcomes of concern were then compared between these two classes. We found that the mean number of work hours completed by students did not differ much from one class to the other. And penalty rates did not increase when research participation was no longer required (a related benefit was that incomplete grades for not satisfying the requirement were no longer necessary). But responses on the credit slips were also similar from one class to the other, which was disappointing because we had hoped that students who participated in research projects to earn extra credit would view their experiences more positively and benefit more from them. Taken altogether, the results suggest that little harm, and perhaps some good, could be done by eliminating the research participation requirement for all the students, as was first proposed. There is still some resistance, however, to making such a dramatic change—resistance caused in part by confusion about how to create comparable extra credit awards across classes taught by instructors with different testing and grading practices, and in part by fears about whether students will indeed continue participating in research projects if they no longer must. I hope that we can resolve this issue sometime soon; otherwise, different instructors may begin to set their own research participation policies rather than following a single departmental policy.

Conclusion

On the whole, using credit slips to evaluate students' research experiences seems to be a valuable practice, one that other departments should consider incorporating into their subject pools. The major disadvantage of this practice is the time and energy required to process large numbers of credit slips, but the resulting access to information about how research participation affects students warrants the effort.

Departments that want to adopt this practice could make the transition easier by starting on a small scale. Credit slips might be introduced, for example, during a semester when enrollments in introductory psychology courses are relatively low, as they often are during the summer. Or, given the apparent stability of students' answers to the questions on our credit slips, it might be sufficient to use such slips only at regular intervals, such as every 3 years, rather than all the time. And there might be other, easier ways to use credit slips, without making them less valuable as sources of information. I welcome suggestions in this regard. In my own department, we have begun to consider a variety of other methods for improving students' research experiences, such as working harder to integrate those experiences into the contents of the introductory psychology courses. This reflects an important truth about subject pools—they are always changing, but never perfect.

References

Diamond, M. R., & Reidpath, D. D. (1992). Psychology ethics down under: A survey of student subject pools in Australia. *Ethics and Behavior, 2,* 101–108.

Lindsay, R. C., & Holden, R. R. (1987). The introductory psychology subject pool in Canadian universities. *Canadian Psychology, 28,* 45–52.

Orne, M. (1962). On the social psychology of the psychological experiment. *American Psychologist, 17,* 776–783.

Sieber, J. E., & Saks, M. J. (1989). A census of subject pool characteristics and policies. *American Psychologist, 44,* 1053–1061.

Wood, J. V. (1989). Theory and research concerning social comparisons of personal attributes. *Psychological Bulletin, 106,* 231–248.

5

Why Do Students Miss Psychology Experiments and What Can Be Done About It?

Darrell L. Butler

One of the most frustrating aspects of research that relies on undergraduate participants is no-shows (i.e., individuals who do not show up for their appointments). Kirkhoff (1990) found that 43% of student experimenters rated no-shows as the worst aspect of their experience as a researcher. Researchers in my department regularly complain to me, the department subject pool coordinator, that undergraduates just do not care and that is why so many do not show up to scheduled research appointments. Motivation could be raised (e.g., by paying students for their time), but the cost to researchers, subject pool administrators, or departments in terms of time, money, or resources could be high. Therefore, researchers and subject pool coordinators need to know how extensive the no-show problem is and the degree to which weak motivation accounts for it.

Thanks to the following people: April Acquino, who suggested using the bogus pipeline and ran some of the subjects in experiment 1; Suzette Hartke, who also ran some of the subjects; William Clark who loaned the physiological recording equipment and trained researchers how to use it; students in the human factors courses who helped in a number of ways; and Paul Biner, Patricia Keith-Spiegel, and Bobbie Rooney for comments on the manuscript.

Several kinds of data suggest that the no-show problem is sizable, at least at some schools. The first kind of evidence comes from subject pool coordinators. I made an extensive analysis of subject pool participation at Ball State University and asked subject pool coordinators at two other large state universities in Indiana to provide no-show data. The analysis of student participation records of more than 15,000 students (i.e., all participants during a 5-year period) at Ball State University indicated a no-show rate of 24%. The subject pool coordinator at Indiana University estimated a no-show rate of 20% (based on tallies from one semester) and the subject pool coordinator at Purdue guessed (no data were analyzed) a no-show rate of 10%. A second kind of evidence was obtained from 20 assistant professors of psychology at a number of universities in the Midwest. They were asked to estimate the no-show rates for the experiments they had run where they had been graduate students. The median estimate of the no-show rate was 20% and none was less than 10%.

Although these rates are high, they are similar to no-show rates of other kinds of institutions. Frankel and Hovell (1978) reported that no-show rates for medical services varied from 20% to 60%. Data on no-show rates at mental health centers are similar. Larson, Nguyon, Green, and Attkinson (1983) reported a no-show rate of 22% for new clients. Turner and Vernon (1976) reported a no-show rate of 29%. Wesch, Lutzker, Frisch, and Dillon (1987) reported a no-show rate of 18%. The average across these studies of mental health centers is 23%. My students and I also surveyed 10 local dentist offices. Receptionists tabulated no-show rates for a 6-month period. As all of the offices called patients to remind them of their appointments, receptionists were asked to tabulate data separately for those they reached by telephone and those they did not reach. For patients not reached by telephone, the no-show rate was 20%.

Lack of motivation is one plausible explanation for these relatively high no-show rates, but there are other reasonable explanations. People may become ill. A variety of illnesses could produce symptoms severe enough that the person would miss appointments. A system designed to reduce no-show rates by affecting motivation probably would have little impact on those who were sick. Another possible reason for missing an appointment is that the person could not find the location within a reasonable period of time. Although this problem probably has only a small effect on no-show rates at most universities, we have found evidence on our campus that some students cannot find some experiment rooms within a reasonable period of time (see Butler, Acquino, Hissong, & Scott, 1993). Steps one would take to reduce this cause of no-shows are different from the ones that traditionally would be used to increase motivation. An additional logical explanation for no-shows is that students forget about their appointments. Although increasing motivation probably could help students remember, the kinds of systems that researchers probably would use to help students remember could be quite different from those most likely to be used to increase motivation.

This chapter reports two experiments concerning why students miss experiments and how researchers can improve the percentage that show up. The first experiment reported was designed to explore reasons students miss experiments and provide estimates of their relative rates of occurrence. We expected lack of motivation to be only one of several factors accounting for the relatively high rate of research appointment no-shows. The second experiment reports an investigation of the impact of reminding students about their appointments.

Experiment 1: Why Students Miss Experiments

Obtaining accurate estimates of the importance of various reasons for missing an experiment appointment is difficult. Students may be hesitant to admit they were apathetic about research. They may believe that apathy is socially undesirable and thus would not want to admit it. Nederhof (1985) defined social desirability as a distortion of responses in a socially desirable direction as a result of self-deception or other-deception. Presumably students can remember if they missed an experiment within the last couple of months, the context surrounding the missed appointment, and the reasons they missed it. In other words, there should be relatively little self-deception. The major research problem is how to reduce possible deception of others, especially researchers trying to investigate the reasons experiments were missed.

One technique that researchers have used to discourage such "lying" is to try to convince subjects that the researcher can tell when they lie. For example, Jones and Sigall (1971) developed the "bogus pipeline." They connected subjects to physiological recording equipment and tried to convince them that the equipment could objectively verify the truth of verbal responses. Millham and Kellogg (1980) have shown that this technique can reduce the other-deception component of social desirability.

Another technique that researchers have used to minimize social desirability biases in verbal responses is to ask people to report about others rather than themselves (e.g., Baird, Noma, Nagy, & Quinn, 1976; Butler & Biner, 1990). The logic of this approach is that people usually have no reason to mislead others about the social desirability of the motives or behavior of anonymous friends and acquaintances. This technique is most useful when the questions concern observable behavior. Its validity is more dubious when the questions concern the thoughts and feelings of others. However, many students talk with friends about going (and not going) to experiments. Thus students have some basis for their beliefs about classmates' reasons for missing experiments. If a student really has no idea about others' reasons, then the student may report his or her own reasons but attribute them to others.

When one attempts to explain the behavior of others, attributions may differ from self-attributions in other ways. A number of studies (e.g., Fiske & Taylor, 1984; Nisbett, Caputo, Legant, & Marceek, 1973) have shown that people have a tendency to use external attributions to explain their own behavior and internal attributions to explain other people's behavior. This actor–observer bias may result from lack of knowledge about others or bias in self-judgment. Determining whether this bias is primarily a distortion of self or others is difficult to establish. Thus this bias casts doubt on the accuracy of self-judgments as well as judgments of others and suggests that some caution should be exercised in interpreting either.

In an effort to reduce or at least measure the effects of various biases, the present experiment involved variants of the two techniques that have been used to reduce social desirability responses. Some subjects were hooked up to machines that measured and recorded heart rate, respiration, and skin conductance. Efforts were made to convince the subjects that the machine could discriminate truth telling from lying. Based on the research described previously, we expected that subjects in this condition would be less likely to provide socially acceptable responses to questions about why they missed experiments and less likely to bias self-ratings in other ways. Other subjects were not connected to any machines but were asked the same questions as those who were. The questions subjects were asked concerned both their own experiment participation and those of their classmates. Based on the research described previously, we expected that subjects would provide less socially accepted explanations for missing experiments when they described classmates than when they described themselves, and that they may be more likely to attribute internal characteristics of classmates as the cause of their missing experiments.

Method

Participants. There were two groups of students from the Department of Psychological Sciences Research Participants Pool. One group, those who would be hooked up to recording equipment, was composed of 51 students who had missed an experiment. The department has a centralized record-keeping system for student participation in research. These students were randomly selected during the middle of two semesters from the population of students (approximately 800 students) who had missed experiments. They were contacted by a researcher in their classrooms (no mention of how they were sampled was provided) and all agreed to participate in this study. The second group, those who would not be hooked up to recording equipment, was composed of 184 other students from the same subject pool. Based on prior no-show data, I expected about 50 of these students to have missed at least one experiment and thus be from the same population as the 51 students in the first group. All participants received course credit for their time. Informed consent was obtained from all subjects and procedures were used to ensure privacy of responses.

Procedure. The procedure was slightly different for the two groups. Subjects in the physiological recording condition were run one at a time. They sat in a padded, wooden chair in a room in which the only other furniture was a physiograph. A Bellows Pneumograph was used to measure respiration, two finger electrodes were connected to the middle fingers of the dominant hand to measure skin conductance, and three steel plated electrodes were placed on the body (each arm and the right leg) to measure heart rate. The subject was given about 10 min to habituate to the apparatus. During this time, the instruments were calibrated. Then the subject was told that the experimenter wanted to verify that the machine was working correctly. The subject was asked to respond truthfully to the question, "What is your name?" The subject was then given a false name and asked to answer the same question with the false name. The printout was removed from the machine and shown to the subject. Differences in the physiological recordings from the two responses were emphasized to increase the subjects' belief that the machine could indicate if they lied. The subjects then were asked a series of questions about their participation in the subject pool:

1. Have you ever missed an experiment?
2. How many have you missed?
3. Why did you miss it?
4. Do you know someone else who missed one? (If not imagine one)

5. Why do you think that person missed the experiment?
6. What would you consider worse, someone who missed an experiment because he or she forgot or someone who was unconcerned and decided not to go?

After answering the questions, subjects were debriefed. During debriefing, all of the subjects stated that they believed the machine could detect truth telling. Researchers explained that it is difficult to determine truth telling from such machines (and why) and that we would not be analyzing the recordings. However, we would be analyzing their answers to the questions.

Participants in the other condition (no physiological recordings) were run in small groups in two classrooms over several days. They were spread out so they could not read materials on each others' desks. They were given a written survey that asked the same questions asked of participants in the physiological recording condition. Participants wrote their responses on the survey.

Results

Participants' stated reasons for missing experiments were categorized by two judges. There were only a few differences in categorizations and they were settled by discussion. Judges identified five major categories of reasons students missed experiments: motivation (e.g., participant just did not feel like going), memory (e.g., participant did not remember until too late), important conflict (e.g., participant was called into work or took a roommate to the hospital), way finding (e.g., participant could not find experiment room), and illness (e.g., participant was at doctor's office). A summary of the percentage of participants who indicated each of these reasons is provided in Table 5-1.

It is quite clear in Table 5-1 that not all reasons are equally likely to be reported by participants. A chi-square goodness of fit was calculated on the frequencies of each reason given

Table 5-1

*Percentage of Subjects Indicating Each Type of Reason
for Missing an Experiment as a Function of
Experimental Conditions*

| Reason | Hooked up[a] | | Not hooked up[a] | | |
	Self[b] ($n = 46$)	Others[b] ($n = 49$)	Self[b] ($n = 69$)	Others[b] ($n = 69$)	Mean
Forgot	43	35	39	36	38
Lack of motivation	22	53	9	30	27
Important conflict	17	8	30	28	22
Illness	11	4	12	3	7
Could not find site	7	0	10	3	5

NOTE: The n's were not equal for the hooked up group because
five subjects stated that they did not miss any experiments and
two could not think of any reasons why others would miss.
[a]Hooked up to physiological recording devices or not.
[b]Judging self or judging others.

for each group assuming equal likelihood of reasons. The chi-
square test indicated that the percentages were not the same
(χ^2 (16) = 132.08, $p < .0001$). Overall, forgetting was the most
commonly indicated reason. Lack of motivation and important conflict were named with moderate frequency. Illness
and way finding problems rarely were indicated.

The percentage of students reporting each reason was different among the various conditions of the study. A chi-
square test of contingency between the reasons and the four
experimental conditions was significant (χ^2 [12] = 41.78,
$p < .001$). The sections that follow explore these differences.

Reasons People Give for Themselves. On the question,
"Why did you miss an experiment?" participants hooked up
to physiological recorders were more likely (22%) than those
not hooked up (9%) to indicate that their reason for missing

an experiment was apathy or lack of motivation (Fisher's exact probability test, $p <. 05$). In contrast, those who were not hooked up were more likely to indicate that they had an important conflict (30%) than students who were hooked up (17%, Fisher's exact probability test, $p < .05$). In other respects, the percentage of reasons provided was similar between these two conditions.

These differences in judgment probably are a result of students' belief that a lack of motivation is socially undesirable. Those who were hooked up were more likely to admit that they were not motivated. Consistent with this hypothesis, 92% of the subjects indicated that apathy or not caring was a much less acceptable reason for missing an experiment than was forgetting.

Judgments of Others. Compared to reasons they gave for themselves, those subjects hooked up were much more likely to indicate that others missed their appointments because they just did not care (51% versus 22%, Fisher's exact probability test, $p < .001$). Subjects who were not hooked up showed a similar bias (30% versus 9%, Fisher's exact probability test, $p < .001$). Subjects were less likely to indicate that other students missed experiments because they were sick or had an important conflict. About half of the subjects indicated that they were thinking of a particular person in answering this question. We compared the percentages for those who were thinking of a specific person and those who were not. The two sets were virtually identical. This finding suggests that this attribution is quite robust and may not be simply a lack of knowledge.

Discussion

This experiment indicates that there are a number of major reasons students miss experiment appointments. A major reason is that they forget. Experiment appointments are not part of their regular schedule and many of these students are doing most of their own scheduling for the first time in their lives. This finding suggests that various systems for reminding students could reduce the no-show rate, and that such reminders could reduce the no-show rate by as much as 40%. Across conditions this estimate is fairly stable (i.e., 35% to 43%). The next experiment was designed to study this possibility.

Another major reason that students miss experiments is that they choose to do something else. Sometimes these other things seemed fairly trivial and judges categorized these responses as apathetic or lacking motivation to show up at their appointment. Sometimes these other things were quite important. For example, judges categorized "taking a very sick roommate to the hospital" or "working because the student's supervisor called them in" as important conflicts. Students who are ill may choose not to attend an experiment. They may decide that it is more appropriate to stay in bed or go to the health center than to go to an experiment. Overall, choosing not to make the appointment accounts for a sizable percentage of no-shows, about 56% across conditions. However, it is unlikely that all of these no-shows can be reduced by providing incentives. Unless incentives were extremely large, they would be unlikely to affect students who had important conflicts or were ill. Based on these results, an incentive program might reduce no-shows up to 25%, although different conditions in this study suggest that this percentage could be anywhere between 9% and 53%.

Another factor accounting for subject no-shows are those subjects who cannot find an experiment. This factor accounted for a very small percentage of no-shows in this experiment. However, if this is a sizable problem on a campus, then clear way-finding systems could be used to alleviate most of this problem (see Butler et al., 1993).

Students in this experiment believed that other students miss appointments primarily because they are apathetic. One cannot help but note the similarity between this finding and the common researchers' belief that most students are apathetic. The causes of this attribution are most likely the same as other examples of the fundamental attribution error or the actor–observer bias. The results of this experiment suggest that this attribution may not be completely justified. Apathy does appear to be a noteworthy reason why some students miss experiments. However, most students appear to miss appointments because they forget, not because they are apathetic.

Experiment 2: Reminding Subjects

Across a number of institutions, there is evidence that reminding people about their appointments can substantially reduce no-show rates. My students and I asked receptionists at 10 local dentist offices to tally no-show rates for 6 months. The no-show rate for patients who received a reminder telephone call was 3% compared to 20% for those not reminded. Turner and Vernon (1976) found that a standardized telephone message reminder reduced the no-show rate at a mental health center from 29% to 13%. Larson et al. (1983) reported that telephone calls from therapists lowered first appointment no-show rates from 22% to 12%. Robert Dailey (personal communication, 1987) reported that using two telephone calls to remind subjects of upcoming counseling research appointments reduced the no-show rate from more than 20% to less than 5%.

The purpose of this experiment was to determine whether reminding subjects of their appointments would reduce the no-show rate to experiments. A secondary goal was to investigate the advantages and disadvantages of different methods of reminding subjects. For this experiment I decided to compare two of the least expensive reminding systems, on-campus mail and local telephone calls.

Method

Participants. A total of 333 undergraduates were selected (the process is described in the procedure section that follows) from those participating in the Department of Psychological Sciences Research Participation Pool. None of these participants had participated in Experiment 1. Based on pilot data, we expected to have more difficulty contacting people by mail. Thus assignment to condition was made randomly with the restriction that the probability for assignment to the mail condition was approximately 40%, whereas it was only approximately 30% for each of the other two conditions. The result was 145 students in the mail condition, 99 in the telephone condition, and 89 in the control condition.

Procedure. On each day for 3 weeks, 20 to 25 students who had signed up for experiments were selected from the various experiments available. Selection included as many different experiments on each day as possible and no more than one person from a page. (Note that each sign up sheet used by students had room for as many as 23 subjects.) Only subjects with appointments at least 3 days away were selected so there would be time to remind them. To keep costs minimal, those subjects assigned to the mail condition were contacted only if they had a campus address in the campus telephone book. On our campus this kind of mail does not have U.S. postal costs. Two or three days before their appointment, they were mailed a slip reminding them of the experiment and asking them to bring the reminder slip with them to the experiment. Those subjects assigned to the telephone condition were contacted only if they had a local telephone number in the campus telephone book. The experimenters attempted to reach them by telephone (a day or two before their appointment) a maximum of two times. If a student was reached, he or she was simply reminded about the experiment and told where it would be and when. No effort was made to contact students in the control condition.

Results

A summary of the show and no-show frequencies is provided in Table 5-2. The control group had a no-show rate of 28%. This rate is similar to the no-show rate in this pool over the last few years (24%).

When students were reminded, the no-show rate was substantially reduced. The no-show rate for students reached by telephone was 12%. This rate is significantly lower than the 28% rate of the control group (Fisher's exact probability test, $p < .02$). Assuming that all students whose reminder was not

Table 5-2

Show and No-Show Frequencies for Subjects in the Telephone
Reminder, Mail Reminder, and No-Reminder Conditions

Condition		Frequency		Percentage
		Showed-up	No-show	No-show
Telephone	Reached	44	6	12
	Not reached	36	13	27
	Total in condition	80	19	19
Mail	Reached	38	0	0
	Unsure if reached[a]	23	10	30
	Not reached	54	20	27
	Total in condition	115	30	21
Control		64	25	28
Total in all conditions		259	74	22

[a]These students did not bring the reminder slip to the research, so we are unsure if they received it.

returned by the postal service did receive it (i.e., both students reached and those we are unsure we reached in the mail condition), the no-show rate for students in the mail condition was 14% (10 of 71), which is significantly lower than the control group no-show rate of 28% (Fisher's exact probability test, $p < .05$). It is unlikely that all of these students received the mailed reminder; however we had no way to estimate what percentage did receive it. Thus we are uncertain if mail led to a lower no-show rate than telephone calls for those who were reached.

Because the percentage of subjects who could be reached by telephone or mail at low cost was fairly low (50% by telephone and a maximum estimate of 49% by mail), the overall impact of reminders was only moderate (20% no-show in reminder conditions versus 28% in the control condition). In the telephone condition, 24% did not have local telephone numbers and 26% were not reached by the second call. In the mail condition, 51% were definitely not reached (i.e., they did not have a campus address or their mail was returned to sender), 26% we know we reached because they brought the reminder card back to us, and the other 23% are unknown. At the end of the semester, we found that a number of the students in the "unknown" category had withdrawn from school; they were no-shows in our study.

Note that no-show rates were 27% for students not reached in the telephone condition and 27% for students not reached in the mail condition. These percentages are similar to the 28% no-show rate for the control condition. If they had been larger than 28%, an alternative explanation would be that they are different populations and that some of the factors that make students unreachable also contribute to students not coming to experiments.

General Discussion

Experiment 2 indicates that reminding students is a useful way to reduce no-shows, but it does not identify a superior method. Local telephone calls and campus mail are inexpensive, but they have two drawbacks. First, the percentage of students reachable by these means may be too low for some campuses. Second, at least for telephone calls, the time required for researchers to contact large groups may more than offset the benefits of reminding. Concern about amount of time could be reduced for mailing reminders if researchers or departments can find a way to have subjects complete their own cards and simplify or automate the mailing procedure. In general, these two technologies may be most useful to researchers running one subject at a time for relatively long periods of time, especially if the researchers have money to pay for postage. In our department, on the first day of classes that are participating in the subject pool, we ask students to put their name, local address, and local telephone number on a 3 × 5 card. These cards are alphabetized and kept in the department office. Researchers who are trying to minimize no-shows can use these cards to locate students. The researchers tell me that this system works very well: They reach at least 80% of the students by telephone or mail.

Other technologies could be used to remind students. Researchers on some campuses may be able to use electronic experiment sign up (e.g., a www registration site) and remind students through e-mail. This solution could be automated, and thus require almost no experimenter or department staff time. However, this solution requires appropriate computer systems and students who regularly use them. There may be few campuses that have both of these assets. However, this may become a viable alternative at campuses in the future.

Although experiment 1 indicated that forgetting was the major cause of no-shows, it also indicated that apathy or lack of motivation was an important cause. An extensive experimental literature demonstrates that the addition of incentives can affect motivation and behavior. For example, Wesch et al. (1987) studied the effect of a small fee on no-shows at a health center. The no-show rate dropped from 18% to 10%.

However, it may be difficult in general to produce such motivation effects in subject pools. In focus group discussions, students generally have told us that although motivation matters, the kinds of "rewards" that departments realistically can provide probably would not be very effective. Of course, researchers with grant money can pay subjects. Otherwise, students argue that experimenters really need to make an effort to make participation convenient and interesting. These are reasonable proposals from students, but I am skeptical that experimenters can always make studies more interesting or convenient. Many faculty who, for example, ask students to complete surveys have indicated that they cannot find ways to make this task highly motivating. However, emphasizing the importance of the information to be gathered may help.

Some skeptics may not be persuaded by these two studies that demonstrate that forgetting may play a larger role in the no-show rate than does apathy. However, the conclusion reached in this set of studies is quite similar to that found in a recent meta-analysis of responses to mail surveys. Yammakino, Skinner, and Childers (1991) found that reminders increased response rates by 31% on the average, whereas incentives only increased response rates by 15% on the average.

Conclusion

This study indicates that forgetting is a major cause of students missing experiments and the no-show rate can be reduced somewhat by using a system to remind students. Motivation is also a major factor, but it is less obvious how researchers can raise motivation in many psychological studies. However, when researchers make the effort to encourage subjects' motivation, there may be many advantages for both students and researchers.

No-show rates vary, but in the present study they were 24% to 28%. These rates are substantial, and are cause for concern. A major reason for students missing experiments is that they forget the appointment. Telephone or mail reminders were shown to reduce no-show rates by 50% or more.

These reminders could be more effective if larger numbers of students were reached. Current addresses and telephone numbers might be obtained by distributing 3 × 5 cards for this purpose at the beginning of the semester. Contacting students by e-mail may be another way to remind students.

Many students who do not show up do so because they have important conflicts or are ill. Reducing no-shows that fall into these categories may be difficult or impossible. Some students may be no-shows because they are unmotivated to attend, and thus choose to do something else. Researchers with grants may be able to provide incentives through paying student participants. Other researchers may be able to develop ways to make participating more interesting or more convenient. A small percentage of students are no-shows because they cannot find the experiment. Way-finding systems could help alleviate this problem.

References

Baird, J. E., Noma, E., Nagy, J. N., & Quinn, J. (1976). Predicted and observed activity patterns in campus settings. *Perceptual and Motor Skills, 43*, 615–624.

Butler, D. L., Acquino, A. L., Hissong, A. A., & Scott, P. A. (1993). Way finding by newcomers in a complex building. *Human Factors, 35*, 159–173.

Butler, D. L., & Biner, P. M. (1990). A preliminary study of skylight preferences. *Environment and Behavior, 22*, 119–140.

Fiske, S. T., & Taylor, S. E. (1984). *Social cognition*. Reading, MA: Addison-Wesley.

Frankel, B. S., & Hovell, M. F. (1978). Health service appointment keeping. *Behavior Modification, 2*, 435–464.

Jones, E. E., & Sigall, M. (1971). The bogus pipeline: A new paradigm for measuring affect and attitude. *Psychological Bulletin, 75*, 349–364.

Kirkoff, K. L. (1990). *The experiences of undergraduate psychological science researchers*. Unpublished honors thesis, Ball State University, Muncie, IN.

Larson, D. L., Nguyon, T. D., Green, R. S., & Attkinson, C. C. (1983). Enhancing the utilization of outpatient mental health services. *Community Mental Health Journal, 10*, 305–320.

Millham, J., & Kellogg, R. W. (1980). Need for social approval: Impression management or self-deception? *Journal of Research in Personality, 14*, 445–457.

Nederhof, A. J. (1985). Methods of coping with social desirability bias: A review. *European Journal of Social Psychology, 15*, 263–280.

Nisbett, R. E., Caputo, C., Legant, P., & Marceek, J. (1973). Behavior as seen by the actor and as seen by the observer. *Journal of Personality and Social Psychology, 27*, 154–164.

Turner, A. J., & Vernon, J. C. (1976). Prompts to increase attendance in a community mental health center. *Journal of Applied Behavioral Analysis, 9*, 141–145.

Wesch, D., Lutzker, J. R., Frisch, L., & Dillon, M. M. (1987). Evaluating the impact of a service fee on patient compliance. *Journal of Behavioral Medicine, 10*, 91–101.

Yammakino, F. J., Skinner, S. J., & Childers, T. C. (1991). Understanding mail survey response behavior: A meta-analysis. *Public Opinion Quarterly, 55*, 613–639.

III

Human Subject Research From an Institutional Perspective

This section is concerned with the interaction between department subject pools and Institutional Review Boards.

Chapter 6 is a case study of the operation of a departmental human subjects committee. Advantages and disadvantages are presented regarding establishing such a committee to evaluate research proposals involving no risk to participants (in lieu of IRB evaluation). The nature of the coordination among the DSP, the IRB, and the Departmental Review Committee is described, as is the way these affect the research participant, the researcher, the administrator, and so forth.

Chapter 7 examines how faculty perceive and interact with IRBs. This chapter reviews subjects' rights, the general IRB review process, recommendations for faculty in negotiating the IRB approval process, and the benefits of IRB participation for the faculty member, including the enhancement of teaching, scholarship, service, and ethics.

6

A Case Study of a Departmental Subject Pool and Review Board

Gregory L. Murphy

A cursory glance at the major psychology journals of 30 to 50 years ago reveals a number of interesting differences between the research activities of psychologists at that time and in the present era. One difference is that empirical research articles usually had a small number of studies reported in each article. In the *Journal of Experimental Psychology*, for example, single- and two-experiment articles were predominant through the 1960s. A less immediately apparent difference is that psychologists often published less in those days. A highly active research psychologist of the 1990s is likely to be an author on four or more articles a year, plus the occasional commentary, book review, or chapter. In the 1960s, such a person would be considered to be an anomaly rather than simply a successful scientist.

The explosion of new journals, plus the increase in size of existing journals, gives clear evidence that more studies are being run in psychology now than ever before. For example,

The writing of this chapter was supported by NIMH grant MH41704. I am grateful to Janet Glaser and Edward Shoben for helpful comments. I especially thank Marti Lanman for patiently instructing me in the details of our human subject committee's operation.

in 1955, the *Journal of Experimental Psychology* (*JEP*) published 850 pages. After splitting into four component journals (plus new journals added after the split, which I am not counting), *JEP* in 1995 totaled 4,040 larger format pages—a five-fold increase at least. Furthermore, since 1955, many new journals have arisen. For example, articles in my own area of research, cognitive psychology, were published primarily in *JEP* in 1955. Since that time, not only has the size of *JEP* increased dramatically, but also newer journals such as *Memory & Cognition*, the *Journal of Memory and Language, Cognition*, and *Cognitive Psychology* have developed into respected outlets, and many of them have also expanded in the past few years.

Based on published papers, it is clear that there has been an explosion of research in psychology over the past few decades. Consequent with that has been an increase in the support needed to do psychological research. Graduate student enrollments, space, equipment, support staff, and grant money have all had to try to keep pace with this increase. In this chapter, I will discuss one particular resource that has also been put under pressure by the increase of psychological research: the use of human subjects. As more psychologists carry out research, and as (I believe) the amount of research carried out by individual psychologists increases, the need for subjects to provide new data has also increased.

The need for subjects creates two primary problems. The first is the need to solicit sufficient subjects to carry out this work. Although some areas of psychology need only a small number of intensively tested subjects (the old joke in sensation research being that the two subjects were the author's left and right eyes), many areas require large numbers of subjects per study. Finding and scheduling these subjects is a nontrivial expense and administrative task. The second problem is the need for adequate ethical review of research. As more studies are carried out, existing review processes can become overloaded. This creates a bottleneck in the research process, which in turn can tempt investigators to avoid seeking ethical review of their work.

This chapter discusses these two issues and ways of addressing them, using the responses of one large psychology department as a possible guide. The first need, that of finding and scheduling subjects, is addressed in part by establishing a computer-based subject pool that is run by the department. The second need, that of adequate ethical review, is addressed by a departmental human subjects committee, which supplements the operation of the Institutional Review Board (IRB). Because a departmental committee is somewhat unusual and may be of particular interest, I will begin by discussing the motivation for and operation of such a committee.

Ethical Review of Psychological Research

Federal regulations for the protection of research subjects require that universities establish an Institutional Review Board to evaluate proposed federally funded research involving human participants (Code of Federal Regulations, Title 45, Part 46, 1991). Institutions receiving federal funds generally must agree that *all* research carried out by their members will meet ethical standards. For nonfederally funded research it may be desirable to establish smaller, department-based human subject committees that ensure ethical standards are upheld. Such "authorized departmental human subjects committees" may have the advantage of providing faster review and may allow different projects to receive ethics reviews than those that are usually sent to an IRB. As a result, a wider range of research subjects may receive protection.

The purpose of the first half of this chapter is to discuss the merits and problems of such departmental systems. I will use the Human Subjects Committee of the Psychology Department at the University of Illinois (UI) at Urbana-Champaign as a case study. This committee, which has been operating for almost 20 years, has developed a variety of procedures and policies that allow smooth operation of proposal evaluation. Drawing on this committee's experience, I will describe some of the difficulties that typically arise in departmental review of research protocols, along with some solutions. Such a committee might not be successful in all circumstances, however, so I will attempt to outline the situations in which departmental committees would be most useful.

Background

The Psychology Department at the University of Illinois (UI) is a large one. The numbers of faculty and graduate students have varied somewhat in recent years, mirroring the university's finances. In 1997–1998 the department had about 57 full-time faculty equivalents and about 190 graduate students, although the latter figure has been as high as 225 in recent years. There were about 1200 undergraduate majors in 1997–1998, and a total of 52,000 instructional units (i.e., credit hours) taught. In addition to undergraduate lecture courses, there is a large number of honors students and undergraduates taking laboratory courses. Thus the department clearly has a critical mass of investigators who could make use of a departmental subject committee.

The UI department is heavily research oriented. Except for some smaller programs, all graduate students are admitted into a PhD program and are expected to carry out research throughout their graduate careers. This applies to clinical students as well, who are active researchers, as well as doing the required practica and clinical training of an APA-accredited program. Some faculty supervise postdoctoral students, and, as I will discuss later, there are also a number of undergraduate students who carry out research projects. In short, the department has more than 200 active researchers, the vast majority of whom use human subjects.

The department is divided up into nine main intellectual and administrative divisions: biological psychology, clinical, cognitive, developmental, industrial/organizational, perception and performance, personality and social ecology, quantitative, and social. As this list suggests, human subjects are used to study a wide variety of research questions. One source of subjects is paid volunteers who sign up on sheets posted around the department for specific experiments. The

main source of subjects is the subject participation component of the introductory psychology course, which provides
a certain number of points toward each student's grade. The
subject pool will be described in more detail later in the chapter.

Decentralized Human Subjects Review

The University of Illinois requires that all research adhere to
the Belmont Principles (The National Commission for the
Protection of Human Subjects of Biomedical and Behavioral
Research, 1978), meet standards of informed consent, minimize any risks to subjects, and protect their privacy and confidentiality. It also requires that *all* research receive some kind
of prior review. The university provides a *Handbook for Investigators: For the Protection of Human Subjects in Research*
(1995), which leaves no doubt about what is covered by its
requirements: "The policy is applicable whether the research
is undertaken on a large or small scale and whether it is
externally funded or not. Pilot projects, student dissertation
and thesis projects, independent study projects, and course
projects must follow this policy if they involve research with
human subjects" (p. 3).

Why such a broad policy? In some institutions, the IRB
handles only the projects that are federally mandated to require review, plus a few others in which investigators seek
approval for their procedures. As a result, a number of
classes of research may not receive a detailed review, including graduate student independent research, undergraduate
class projects, pilot work that has not yet been funded, and
unfunded research by faculty investigators. However, an argument can be made that it is exactly these projects that most
need institutional review. Federal grant panels are asked to
consider the treatment of participants in proposed research
as part of their evaluation, and thus funded research is typically reviewed by experts in the field in addition to the IRB
review. Furthermore, faculty members submitting grants on
a certain topic are very likely to have had experience in car-

rying out research in this area and would therefore be aware of the prevailing standards and practices in the field. In contrast, undergraduates and beginning graduate students are unlikely to be familiar with these practices. Having had less experience in designing and running studies, students can be insensitive to ethical issues. They may not realize that some subjects would be upset by a procedure they plan to use (e.g., deception, presenting depictions of violence). They will not have had experience in writing adequate consent and debriefing forms. They may not understand the importance of keeping sensitive information confidential. In short, undergraduates and beginning graduate students may be the people whose projects are *most* in need of ethical review.

As one can imagine, however, a university IRB could easily become swamped with such projects. Suppose that a psychology department requires its students to take a laboratory class of some kind, and that three such classes require students to do final projects in which they collect some data. If the students each submitted a proposal to the university IRB, then it might receive 50 to 200 proposals a year just from this one requirement (depending on the size of the department). Students doing independent study, honors research, graduate first-year projects, master's theses, and so on would all add to this figure. This rapidly increasing number of proposals is the reason that many departments do not provide an independent review of undergraduate proposals or other forms of unfunded research. In some cases, there is a minimal form of review, in which a course (e.g., a lab course) receives a blanket approval for its activities, and the instructor is expected to ensure that the projects are ethical.

Lack of review of student proposals cannot be completely attributed to the amount of work that would be required on the part of the IRB. It can be a considerable amount of effort for an instructor to help prepare the proposals for an entire class of students who have never done this before. Even supervising a couple of honors students in this task can take considerable time. Furthermore, many IRBs meet on a monthly basis. Thus it is necessary for the students to meet a very strict deadline to get their proposals reviewed on time.

If the student's roommate becomes ill or the printer breaks the night before the proposal is due (extremely common events, in my experience), resulting in a missed deadline, then the proposal is simply not reviewed. If changes to the proposal are required, then another month may elapse before it can be reviewed again. A month's delay may be prohibitive within the context of a semester-long course or even for a year-long honors project. So there are many practical problems that make it difficult to review student projects, from the perspectives of the student, the instructor, and the IRB.

Thus one advantage of a departmental committee would be to deal with student proposals. As I will discuss, such a committee would typically be more timely and flexible. Arrangements could be made in advance to review the proposals from a course, or to return all proposals involved in masters projects by a given deadline. And because each committee would handle proposals from only one department, the potentially large number of student proposals would be somewhat reduced. Unlike a university IRB, a psychology department committee would not handle proposals from the medical school, anthropology, sociology, the education school, kinesiology, and so forth, in addition to psychology.

The next sections of this chapter discuss how such a committee might be constituted, as well as some of the restrictions on its operations. This discussion cannot be taken as a universal set of recommendations, however, because any such committee must be consistent with the policies of one's university, including its assurance to the federal government on human subjects review. In particular, if the university has said in its assurance that *all* research using human subjects will be reviewed by the IRB then a department could not set up its own committee. (It is possible to set up a number of IRBs within a single institution, and some large research universities do so. However, each one would have to follow strictly the federal regulations involving membership and meetings, which are sometimes inconsistent with the advantages of a departmental committee.)

General Goals of a Departmental Subject Committee

A departmental subject committee should have the goal of reviewing proposed research for ethical treatment of human subjects in a complete and timely manner. The standards that the committee applies should generally be those that the university IRB would apply to federally funded research, even if this is not legally required (and it may be). I would argue that it is wise to use the same standards as the IRB does for two reasons. First, from the perspective of the subject it makes no difference whether a study is a federally funded project or is locally funded or unfunded. The source of funding does not seem relevant to ethical standards. Nonetheless, we have found that some investigators feel that a departmental committee should be more lax than the IRB. The idea seems to be that the departmental committee is kind of a junior IRB, with fewer rules, fewer responsibilities, and lower standards. But although the committee would certainly prefer fewer duties, subjects' rights would not be protected by weaker standards.

Perhaps these investigators feel that the federal standards are overly stringent, and so they prefer to establish weaker requirements in cases in which federal standards are not mandated. That argument brings us to the second reason for having consistent standards, namely issues of legal liability. If a subject is injured, is psychologically damaged, or is simply very unhappy with his or her experience in a study, the investigators and university may be subject to legal action. Clearly, the defense against such action will be more difficult if the work has been evaluated by rules that do not meet the federal standards. It will be difficult for a university to explain why it requires some research to have a consent form, while other research that seems extremely similar is not required to have one; or to justify why parental consent is obtained for IRB-approved studies but not department-approved studies. Such differences give an impression of inadequate review at the departmental level, whereas applying the same standards at all levels would allow one to point out that the federal guidelines were followed in approving the study in question, even if they were not legally required.

Another goal of a departmental committee is to provide faster service than one usually receives from an IRB. At UI, investigators can turn in proposals to the departmental committee whenever they are ready (there is no waiting for the beginning of the month), and they are logged in and reviewed immediately. Although we tell investigators that they cannot expect an answer in less than a week (given the vicissitudes of faculty schedules), in the vast majority of cases the response time is in fact less than a week. However, such a response time is only possible when there is a simple procedure for evaluating proposals and when there is administrative support for communicating with the committee and investigator. As will be described later, it is probably not possible to achieve such service while following the usual IRB administrative practices. However, it is certainly possible to apply the same standards that an IRB would, using different review procedures.

Another possible advantage is that a departmental subject committee may be able to provide a more expert review of a given topic. A proposal by clinical psychologists can be reviewed by someone who is also a clinical researcher; a memory experiment can be evaluated by a cognitive psychologist. Not only will this allow the committee to identify possible problems, it may allow it to make concrete suggestions about how to resolve them. Someone who has faced similar problems in his or her own research may be able to draw on these experiences to help modify a consent form or suggest an alternate procedure.

Finally, the departmental human subject committee may agree to take on other responsibilities that an IRB is not responsible for. The UI Psychology Department committee evaluates all studies that propose to use the departmental subject pool. As described in some detail later, the committee evaluates each experiment for its appropriateness for this pool and gives advice on how to make the experiment a valuable educational experience. This is part of the committee's educational mission, which is not part of the IRB mission.

Determining What a Departmental Committee Can Handle

As mentioned earlier, government regulations specify that most grant proposals using human subjects be reviewed by the university IRB. Thus this research cannot be approved by a departmental committee. A further restriction that UI applies to its departmental committees, which seems advisable in general, is that they review only research that involves no more than minimal risk. Departmental committees may not have the breadth of membership, including nonscientists from the community, which is advisable when making judgments about the risk–benefit ratio of a study. The majority of research done in most psychology departments is in the minimal risk category—that is, risk that is no greater than that encountered in the subject's everyday life. When research involves physiological interventions or medical or psychological treatments, it is best to receive an evaluation from the university IRB.

The departmental committee can handle class projects, proposals by undergraduates, thesis and other graduate research, and work by faculty. It is probably desirable to limit proposals to those that originate from members of the department, as people in other departments that do not have such a committee might wish to avail themselves of the faster turnaround time of the departmental committee rather than go to the university IRB. Not only will this increase the workload of committee members, it is possible that they do not have the expertise necessary to evaluate this work. If experimental psychologists staff the committee, they may not realize the possible problems involved in research in anthropology or education. The university IRB that attempts to have broad representation across different disciplines is better equipped to deal with such protocols.

Administration of the Departmental Review Process

In this section, I will describe as a case study the operations of the UI Psychology Department committee. The procedures, forms, and rules that are used have been developed over a number of years of practice, and so they work quite smoothly by now. However, some problems are also known that cannot be easily remedied without changing the entire system. I am not claiming that the UI's system is the only possible one or even the best one. It may be that departments that are smaller or have different research activities could use a very different structure successfully. However, I would strongly recommend that any committee develop standard forms and procedures for review rather than using a more informal system (e.g., a colleague describes the study to another colleague, who then verbally approves it). The paperwork of the formal system allows an objective statement of what was proposed and approved, which would come in handy if there is ever a question about the study. Also, the use of "official" forms reinforces the point that this is an important enterprise that all parties should take seriously. Although there is considerable (boring) administrative work involved in setting up the procedures and record keeping involved in a more formal system, I believe that this system is more likely to be effective in the long run.

In my department, the Human Subjects Committee is constituted of faculty members from a variety of different areas of psychology that test human subjects. In addition, the instructors of the introductory psychology course, the subject pool coordinator, and a member of the computer support staff are ex-officio members. Review of research is only done by the faculty members, although the entire committee may be consulted on matters of policy and changes in procedures.

The committee meets at the beginning of the year to review the policies and ensure that similar standards are being applied by all members. Any changes in policy from previous years are discussed, and if members have developed any concerns as a result of proposals they have reviewed, these are also aired at this time. This meeting is important, because most of the operation of the committee during the year does not involve meetings, which is the major factor in ensuring a quick response.

The department supports a full-time secretary who coordinates the subject pool (described in more detail later) and who also is responsible for maintaining records, logging in protocols, and communicating to investigators and committee members. In most departments, a full-time position would not be necessary. A secretary or administrative assistant can do the necessary paperwork and maintain the records as the need arises—probably only for a few hours each week. (In fact, most of our coordinator's activity is taken up with administering the subject pool, which involves more than 1000 students each semester. Review of proposals can be time consuming at a few peak periods in the semester but is usually less demanding.)

Every semester, department members (faculty, graduate students, postdocs, and visitors) receive written reminders that every study needs prior approval. Although redundant to many, these notices ensure that everyone is aware of the policy, especially new students and visitors.

Past experience has shown that an unstructured submission procedure often leads to incomplete proposals. As a result, the department has developed a five-page form that asks a series of questions about the project. The first issue is to identify the investigator and his or her status (faculty, student, or visitor). All research must be overseen by a responsible faculty investigator who accepts responsibility for the ethical conduct of the research. Questions about the subjects to be used and the means of soliciting them follow. Investigators indicate the method of informed consent to be used by checking one of five alternatives. Similar checklists ask about procedures to ensure the confidentiality or anonymity of data collection, whether there is any deception, and how debriefing will be accomplished. Such checklists are easier for the committee to interpret than the investigator's own descriptions, which are often incomplete. Finally, the responsible faculty member is asked to sign a statement indicating that departmental and university guidelines will be followed.

In addition to the form, investigators submit a description of the study's methods. If necessary, a justification of the study as being of minimal risk is given. The protocol must include the consent and debriefing forms. If verbal consent is used, then the protocol must indicate in detail what subjects will be told to obtain consent. A number of investigators are not completely familiar with all the required parts of a consent form. As a result, we supply a general description of the required parts, as well as a sample, so that investigators may simply copy preapproved language as appropriate. A similar description and sample is used for the debriefing form. Although detailed debriefing may not be required as part of the ethical review, it is part of our educational mission.

The protocol is given to the staff member who coordinates the committee's activities, who then assigns it to a committee member. The members of the committee are all familiar with the university and departmental regulations. Furthermore, a large amount of specific "case law" has arisen over the years that is known by the committee at large—some of it being reviewed during the meeting at the beginning of the year. This case law is a set of precedents of the sort that taking electroencephalographs (EEGS) is considered a minimal risk procedure, but PET scans (Positron Emission Tomography) are not. For the vast majority of cases with well-known and simple procedures, a meeting of the entire committee is not necessary. One does not need to schedule a meeting of six faculty members to determine that the consent form does or does not include a statement that subjects may withdraw from the experiment. When a proposal has the usual sorts of problems (or does not appear to have any problems), it is simply handled by the committee member who initially receives it. This accounts for the speed in handling the typical proposal. Of course, new situations do arise, especially for a new committee member who may not yet be familiar with the "case law." In such a circumstance, the member consults with the committee head, who knows the past policies. When the situation is truly original, or if an investigator objects to a decision by the initial reviewer, then the entire committee becomes involved in the decision. In the past, this required a meeting, which could take quite some time to schedule. Nowadays, such a decision is most likely to be made over electronic mail, unless it involves a major change in policy or an extremely complex problem. For example, the committee recently decided over e-mail that the risk of being bitten by a tarantula (even of a nonpoisonous variety) was not one normally encountered by our subject population in everyday life. No meeting seemed necessary to discuss this.

The committee member reads the proposal form, the description of the study, and other materials supplied by the investigator. The member may make one of three decisions: *approved, disapproved,* or *tentative approval.* The first two are self-explanatory; tentative approval is used when a point needs clarification or when there are only minor errors that need fixing. For example, if a consent form is missing a standard line, the reviewer might decide to give the protocol tentative approval, which becomes full approval when the corrected consent form arrives. Similarly, the reviewer might make a comment such as, "I assume that the subjects will all be 18 or older. If this is correct, then the project is approved. If not, then the consent procedure for minors must be described and justified." If the study in fact has only adult subjects, then the investigator would reply that this is the case, and the project would not undergo further review.

In many cases, the protocol has one or two possible problems rather than any serious ethical concern. The reviewer would describe these problems, which are then transmitted to the investigator, with a "disapproved" decision. The investigator prepares a revised proposal, which is then given to the same committee member for review (along with the old proposal and the comments). Such revisions can usually be checked in a few minutes, and so the turnaround time is often only a day.

The subject pool coordinator retains files of the proposals and committee reviews. Approval of a project is good for one year, at which time experimenters are asked whether the project is still being carried out. If so, and if there are no changes to it, the approval is extended for another year. At the end of this period, investigators must reapply for approval. In the past, approvals had been renewed indefinitely often, without a full review being required. However, this practice can lead to drift, as investigators make slight changes to their procedure with every experiment, eventually resulting in a procedure that is quite different from the original one that was approved years ago. Furthermore, as regulations sometimes change, a study that was approved 5 years ago may not be in compliance with the existing rules (e.g., the consent form may require updating). A 2-year period is a compromise between ensuring maximum compliance and not overloading investigators with paperwork. The subject coordinator reminds investigators of projects that are about to expire, as faculty seldom remember such matters on their own.

The record-keeping activity is necessary for the department to ensure that all studies have been properly reviewed. As suggested earlier, such records can also be important to safeguarding the investigator or the department if there is ever a question about the treatment of subjects in a study. If the investigator can show that he or she was strictly following the procedures that were approved, that will in part document that the investigator was taking ethical concerns seriously. In contrast, if an investigator has done something that is unethical or inappropriate, the department may be able to show that it never approved this project, or that the approved project differed from what was actually carried out. For these reasons, the UI Psychology Department retains records of proposals for at least 3 years after the end of the study, as does the university IRB.

In addition to the usual ethical concerns that any IRB would address, the UI Psychology Department subject committee also ensures that subjects from the introductory psychology pool receive an educational experience. Although such judgments are made at the same time as the ethical review, the next section reviews this issue separately, as rather different considerations are involved.

Departmental Subject Pool

Subjects in psychology department research at UI come from one of three main sources: the introductory psychology subject pool, sign-up sheets placed around campus, and solicitation of off-campus populations. For many researchers, the departmental subject pool is the largest source of subjects. This is especially true for those who work in areas that require large numbers of subjects: social psychology, personality, and individual differences in general. A number of researchers in the department study group processes, which requires very large numbers of participants. Because grant support is not always available to pay subjects, the departmental subject pool is an important source of subjects for these researchers.

Of course, the need for subjects does not justify a class requirement. Our rationale is that becoming involved in research as a subject provides an educational experience of hands-on research done at the cutting edge of psychology, an experience that is not easily obtained in the classroom. (Our introductory class is not a laboratory course, which makes hands-on experience as a subject especially valuable.) The question of the educational value of subject requirements has received considerable attention, and I will not address it here. (For example, Coulter [1986] and Sieber & Saks [1989] argue that subjects do not feel that they have learned much from their participation, whereas Landrum & Chastain [1995] find that subjects value their research experience. See other chapters in this volume for a discussion of these issues.) I will instead address some of the specific mechanisms by which the subject pool operates, and the ways in which the UI department tries to maximize the student's educational experience.

Subjects are required to complete up to 6 hours of research experience during the semester-long course. In reality, each "hour" is 50 minutes long, as subjects must be released 10 min before class time. The size of the introductory class is quite large, varying from about 1200 to 2500 students per semester. As a result of the variation in enrollment, the number of subject hours in a given semester ranges from about 7000 to 14,000. The system is therefore somewhat involved, and to structure my description of it, I present it from three perspectives: that of the student, that of the investigator, and that of the administrator.

The Student's Perspective

The subject pool is introduced to students in their extensive class syllabus and is discussed by the instructor on the first day of class. (It is also mentioned in the course catalog.) This ensures that students know the class requirements at the beginning of the semester, and it also increases the chance that they will correctly carry out their part in the process. An alternative exercise is available for the few students who do not wish to participate as subjects. During the first few days of classes, students fill out a schedule card, indicating when they are free to perform experiments. They also provide other information, such as their gender, handedness, whether they are native speakers of English, and whether they have any disabilities that might interfere with doing an experiment. This information is rather laboriously entered into a database by part-time office workers, who type in each student's schedule. Such a process could no doubt be computerized, using standard test forms for data entry, and such an improvement is likely to happen in the next few years. Alternatively, any university that has an easily accessible computer network could have students submit their own schedules over the network.

Because of the adding and dropping of courses at the beginning of the semester, as well as the start-up time involved in entering students' schedules, experiments do not begin until the third full week of the semester. Approximately 10 days prior to a scheduled experiment, students receive a mailed notification of their participation in that study. However, given the uncertainties of campus mail, this information is supplied redundantly. Lists are posted every week at various locations in the Psychology Building that give the time and location of every subject's assignment to an experiment. Students are reminded by their instructors to check the assignments on a weekly basis. Furthermore, such lists are now made available on computer, via the "gopher" information retrieval system. The Psychology Department maintains a gopher database, and the assignments for each week are kept as separate files. Thus students can check on whether they have been assigned to experiments from home or while they are on a university workstation; this information is available 24 hours a day. It may be possible to eliminate the mailing of notices when regular computer use becomes truly universal (and highly reliable).

Although students are scheduled for experiments only during the times they have marked as free on their schedules, there are inevitably temporary conflicts or schedule changes that arise from time to time. It is the student's obligation to call and cancel the experiment by contacting either the experimenter (whose number is listed on the notification) or the subject coordinator in order to receive a "notified absence." If subjects do not call in advance, they are given an "unnotified absence" for that session. Each student is allowed one unnotified absence without penalty. However, if two such absences occur, then the student is dropped from the subject pool (though he or she still receives credit for experiments that were completed). When a true emergency arises that would prevent a student from notifying the experimenter, a notified absence can be given instead. If a subject has consistently cancelled sessions, even with sufficient warning to avoid an unnotified absence, he or she must fulfill the obligation during a make-up session that is held at the end of the semester. Thus there is no penalty for notified absences, but students are expected to make up the participation at a later time—either through being assigned to a new experiment, or in the make-up session.

The Investigator's Perspective

The subject pool involves a certain amount of paperwork on the part of the investigator, but this is outweighed by a number of advantages over popular alternatives, such as soliciting paid subjects and subject pools in which students sign up on posted schedules of each experiment. Experimenters request a certain number of subject hours at the beginning of the semester. Once they receive their allocation (through a process described in the next section), they may request subjects. Experimenters hand in a form listing the number of subjects they wish at a given time. They may request subjects of a certain type—classified by the information listed on the student's schedule sheet. For example, an investigator might want groups of three women half the time and groups of three men the other half; or he or she may want only native English speakers for a study of syntactic processing; or no restrictions may be requested.

After making the request, the investigator has only to wait for the subjects to arrive at the requested time. A week to 10 days in advance, a list of the subjects who were selected to be in the study is mailed to the investigator. It may be that no subject of a given description could make it at one or more of the requested hours (the available subjects may have already been scheduled for a different study). This happens seldom through the middle of the semester, but increasingly often toward the end, as more and more subjects complete their requirement. Because the subjects themselves are notified by mail and by the posting of assignments, the investigator does not need to do anything further. Some investigators choose to contact subjects the day before to remind them of their appointment, but this is not required. Once the subject has completed the session, the investigator checks the student's name off on the list of subjects, which is returned to the subject pool coordinator. This information is entered into the computer to keep track of absences and completed sessions.

One advantage of this system is the random assignment of subjects to experiments (within the constraints requested by the experimenter). That is, unlike sign-up sheets and other methods of contacting subjects, there is no self-selection involved in deciding to participate in the experiment. Of course, a student can decide not to participate in the experiment once he or she finds out what it is about—consent forms all mention this—but this happens very seldom, as all of the studies are of no more than minimal risk. (If a student objects to being in a particular study, he or she simply reenters the pool to become eligible for a different one.) As a result, a student who might not sign up for a study of perception or of group decision making will now be exposed to this research. And experimenters who may have been reaching a biased sample of subjects through advertising for subjects will have greater breadth in their pool. Of course, there is still the fact that all of the students are taking introductory psychology, but given the size of the course, a random selection from this pool seems to be more representative of the student body than most other methods of soliciting subjects. So, in addition to any practical benefits of using the subject pool, the random selection may be providing better samples.

In short, the procedure is very simple: The request is sent in and the subjects arrive. Of course, things can become more confusing in some exceptional cases, but it is a simple system from the perspective of the investigators.

The Administrator's Perspective

One reason that the system is simple for investigators is that the subject coordinator's office does most of the paperwork and scheduling. Fortunately, most of these activities are now performed by computer, such as the assignment of subjects to specific experiments. The computer also generates notices to be mailed to the students at the same time. Nonetheless, some labor is necessary in sending out the announcements, entering data, and dealing with problems.

At the beginning of the semester, faculty, graduate students, undergraduate honors students, and postdocs may all request hours. These requests are tabulated, and a standard procedure is followed to derive an allocation for each person. The procedure that my department has found works best is as follows. First, we overallocate the number of hours by 35%—for example, if there are 10,000 subject hours available in one semester, we actually allocate 13,500 to investigators. If one gives out exactly the same number of hours as are truly available, any investigator who does not use all of his or her allocation would be depriving a student of the opportunity of completing the requirement. Also, those hours might have been used by another investigator who used up her entire allocation. We allocate more hours than are truly available, which means that if an individual investigator cannot complete a study that semester, the subject pool is not disrupted.

This 135% of the hours is now divided into three general pools: priority, faculty, and student allocations. According to departmental policy, students who are using subjects to fulfill a degree requirement (an MA, PhD, or honors thesis) are given their full request, before any other hours are allocated (hence the name "priority" allocation). This policy was adopted to avoid a possible situation in which students are required by their committees to do three studies for their master's thesis and yet are not given resources to carry out these studies. There is, of course, a limit on the number of hours that any individual student can request for each priority purpose: 200 subject hours for the MA, 300 for the PhD. The faculty pool, which includes postdocs as well, is allocated 70% of the remaining hours. Students doing independent study projects receive 30% of the nonpriority hours. Faculty are given more hours largely because their work is often in collaboration with students anyway, and so students benefit from their allocations.

Within each of the nonpriority pools (faculty and students), hours are allocated according to an exponential formula. This formula (developed by Professor Edward Shoben) results in small requests being almost completely filled. Larger requests get an increased number of hours, but this increase gets smaller and smaller as the size of the request increases. The exact formula for deriving each investigator's allocation is as follows:

$$\text{Amount allocated} = \lambda(1 - exp[-\text{amount requested}/\lambda])$$

where λ is a parameter that depends on the number of hours available, and *exp* is the exponential function. This formula is applied to every request to derive its allocation. As can be seen, the parameter λ is the maximum amount that anyone can receive. The formula has the nonobvious property that the amount allocated will never exceed the amount requested, even when the request is much smaller than λ. For example, if λ = 100, and a request were for 50 hours, the number allocated would be 39 hours; if λ = 1000, the number allocated would be 49 hours. The size of λ is determined by the subject pool coordinator using the allocation program in an interactive manner. She tries larger and smaller values of this parameter until the allocations for each investigator sum to the total number of hours to be allocated. The parameter is larger in semesters with many subject hours available.

As a result of this process, in a typical spring semester (the lower enrollment semester), a faculty member requesting 100 hours might receive 93 of them; someone requesting 200 hours might receive 120 of them; someone requesting 500 might receive 122. The reason for such a formula is to allow every investigator access to some reasonable number of subjects. If the number of allocated subjects were a linear function of the number of requested subjects, then large requests would take away hours from small requests. For example, if every investigator received 50% of his or her request, then someone who requested 500 hours would get 250 subjects, but someone who wanted only 20 to run a small study would get only 10, which seems rather inequitable. The exponential formula is roughly linear for small requests, but at some point, the function flattens out, so that even very large requests do not get appreciably more hours (e.g., the function in the example above has flattened out near 125). There is also a limit on the largest possible request to prevent investigators from asking for 100,000 hours, which would have an adverse effect on the pool, even with the exponential formula.

Once the allocations have been assigned, the subject pool coordinator sends out information about requesting subjects. The request forms are due weekly, and a student employee types the requests into the computer. These requests are filled by the computer, as described previously, which also generates the student notices and list of subjects for each week, sent to the investigators. When investigators return their lists, the student employee uses the computer again to mark the student as having completed the session, having an excused absence, or not having appeared.

At the end of the semester, there are always some students who have had a number of excused absences and as a result have not received many points for the requirement. These subjects may take part in a final make-up session. The make-up session is organized by the subject coordinator without the benefit of the computer. The "reading day" between the end of classes and final exams is often used for this purpose. Usually, three or four consecutive hours in the afternoon and evening are designated for this purpose. Subjects sign up for as many experiments as they need to fulfill their requirement. Because all subjects are run in such a short time, these sessions are used primarily for questionnaires, group testing, or other large-number sessions.

Evaluation of the System

Many of the advantages and disadvantages of this system would be common to any system in which students perform research as part of a course requirement or to receive extra credit, and therefore I will not dwell on those particular issues. The disadvantages of this sort include subjects whose attitudes range from enthusiastic to hostile, lack of control over the basic population (which is determined by course registration), overrepresentation of first- and second-year students, and a persistent feeling that subjects become inattentive toward the end of the semester (in spite of evidence to the contrary; Cooper, Baumgardner & Strathman, 1991; Langston, Ohnesorge, Kruley & Hasse, 1994). The advantages of a course-based system are primarily the guarantee of a subject population semester after semester, at low cost. The educational benefits to the students vary, I believe, with their decision about whether to take an active part in the experience. Some students simply wish to get back to their other activities as quickly as possible and do not read the debriefing form or talk to the researcher. Others ask many questions and find the experience to be interesting as well as educational. Just as some students do not pay attention to lectures or do the assigned reading, some do not take advantage of the possibility of learning from a research experience. Nonetheless, we continue to give lectures and assign readings, and the best students do seem to learn from these experiences as well as from research participation.

The particular advantages of the more complex computer-based system that I have described are considerable. First, the random assignment of subjects to studies allows investigators to rule out any self-selection bias that might affect the choice of subjects in their experiment (though, of course, the status of subjects as college students is another issue). Second, the automatic scheduling of the computer system takes an enormous burden off investigators who do not have to contact and schedule individual subjects. This is also simpler for the subjects, who receive mailed and posted notification of their assignments, rather than having to sign up or be available for telephone contact to complete their scheduling.

The disadvantages are primarily those of the initial set-up of the system. The computer programs must be written, and they must be capable of handling a large database of students, their schedules, the studies they have completed, and so on. It may be that a standard database program could be used to store all this information, and then be accessed by the subject coordinator on a weekly basis. Our own program allows a more automatic operation, which required greater initial programming time but involves less work on a weekly basis. Using any kind of automatic system places constraints on how quickly subjects can be obtained. In our system, there is a two-week lag between the request of subjects and when they arrive. This is necessary to notify subjects of their appointment in plenty of time. The simpler sign-up sheet system can be more flexible in that if one decides on Monday to run 10 more subjects, one can put up a scheduling sheet to have them all come in on Wednesday (if they notice the new sign-up sheet, if they decide to sign up, etc.).

A final issue, which can be seen as either an advantage or disadvantage, is that a computer-based system is run by a central administrator rather than by individual investigators. Faculty do not worry about whether subjects will appear, or how to contact them, and so on. However, the department must provide the central administrator. This might be a staff member who takes on this job in addition to other duties, or it might be someone who is connected with the introductory psychology course (a teaching assistant, for example). Whether budgets allow the use of office personnel for this purpose (including the initial programming and set-up) is something that each department must decide on its own. Another possibility is for researchers with external funding to contribute something to the salary of this administrator in order to have access to the subject pool for their funded projects. Alternatively, one could argue that the department should cover this administrative duty from indirect recovery costs from grants.

Conclusion

Unless and until research activity in psychology decreases (a prospect that has some champions—see Hunt, 1995), there will be increasing demand for the ethical evaluation of psychological research. For minimal-risk research, a departmental human subjects committee provides a number of advantages. It may encourage ethical review of student proposals or unfunded work that is not presently being reviewed by the IRB. The prospect of faster, more informed reviews is certainly an attractive one. At the same time, of course, it is necessary to ensure that the standards of the committee do not fall prey to cronyism or bias.

With the advent of powerful desktop computers, it is increasingly feasible for departments to set up computerized databases for scheduling subjects. There is still some human labor involved in this process, in entering subjects' initial schedules and their participation data. However, as computer networks become ever more prevalent, it may be possible to spin off even these functions to the students and investigators themselves. Such a system has a number of advantages over class solicitation and sign-up sheets, and it seems likely that these systems will become more the rule than the exception in the future.

References

Cooper, H., Baumgardner, A., & Strathman, A. (1991). Do students with different characteristics take part in psychology experiments at different times of the semester? *Journal of Personality, 59,* 109–127.

Coulter, X. (1986). Academic value of research participation by undergraduates. *American Psychologist, 41,* 317.

Handbook for investigators: For the protection of human subjects in research. (1995). Urbana: University of Illinois at Urbana-Champaign.

Hunt, E. (1995). Swan song. *Journal of Experimental Psychology: General, 124,* 347–351.

Landrum, R. E., & Chastain, G. (1995). Experiment spot-checks: A method for assessing the educational value of undergraduate participation research. *IRB: A Review of Human Subjects Research, 17,* 4–6.

Langston W., Ohnesorge, C., Kruley, P., & Haase, S. J. (1994). Changes in subject performance during the semester: An empirical investigation. *Psychonomic Bulletin & Review, 1,* 258–263.

The National Commission for the Protection of Human Subjects of Biomedical and Behavioral Research. (1978). *The Belmont Report: Ethical principles and guidelines for the protection of human subjects of research* (DHEW Publication No. OS 78-0012). Washington, DC: U.S. Government Printing Office.

Sieber, J. E., & Saks, M. J. (1989). A census of subject pool characteristics and policies. *American Psychologist, 44,* 1053–1061.

The Why, What, How, and When of Effective Faculty Use of Institutional Review Boards

Janet F. Gillespie

Writers in the area of research ethics (e.g., Rosnow, Rotheram-Borus, Ceci, Blanck, & Koocher, 1993) have noted that researchers in psychology have, over the past 20 years or so, faced ever greater strictures and limitations on the ways in which they may conduct research. Guidelines for the development and design of psychological experiments, as well as data collection and analysis and dissemination of research findings, are now explicit and federally mandated (Rosnow et al., 1993).

The recent origin of these guidelines can be traced to the release of the Belmont Report in 1978, which was the first U.S. government publication to articulate explicit rules for all human subject research conducted in academic, medical, and military settings (National Library of Medicine, 1986a). The Belmont Report led to creation of the federal government's Office for Protection from Research Risk (OPRR), a division of the Department of Health and Human Services (DHHS). OPRR mandates are today implemented and enforced at the university level by Institutional Review Boards (IRBs). IRBs are also referred to as *review committees for human participant research, research review boards, ethics boards,* or sometimes simply the *human subjects committee.*

Research universities should always have an IRB, but colleges that are primarily undergraduate institutions may or may not have an IRB or a detailed procedure for review of research. Similarly, community colleges, whose mission is more teaching than research, will typically not have an IRB either. A member of a university faculty, or any college student who does any research, will soon learn that all research involving human participants must be reviewed by the IRB before any participants are recruited or data collected. Specific types of projects this pertains to include all faculty research, graduate students' master's theses and doctoral dissertations, senior theses, and undergraduate honors projects. IRB review also extends to undergraduates' class term projects if data are collected, even class opinion surveys in which one gathers information from one's peers and classmates about any topic. IRB review is also necessary in the case of professors handing out personality measures in class, having their students complete them and then learn to score the measures by analyzing their own responses. It applies to graduate students' recruiting friends for intellectual testing to allow "practice" administration of tests for courses in psychological assessment. In summary, the domain of governance of campus IRBs is quite broad.

This chapter will review ways in which college faculty may effectively negotiate the institutional review board review process and learn from it for their own benefit and that of their students, clients, and the research participants with whom they will interact. It is written with practical suggestions in mind, and suggestions for "best practice" for ethical, safe and meaningful research. Included are the following topics: (a) contemporary "subjects' rights" initiatives and the history of IRBs; (b) IRB roles and responsibilities and criteria IRBs must follow in evaluating a research project as ethical and scientific; (c) the IRB review process—steps and assignment of category of "risk"; (d) recommendations for negotiating the IRB approval process, including steps in completing a standard IRB proposal and caveats to note, including common faculty "pitfalls" in interactions with IRBs; and (e) IRB functions and benefits for the faculty member—the IRB process as a learning experience for teaching, scholarship, service, and ethics.

Contemporary Subjects' Rights Initiatives and the History of IRBs

Modern scientific research has for the most part relied almost entirely on the integrity of the investigator to guarantee patients' rights; IRBs are a recent development (Rosnow et al., 1993). This reliance on the individual was successful in some cases, and professionals did accomplish vital medical research while using adequate precautions to protect their patients (National Library of Medicine, 1986b). An example is the pioneering yellow fever interventions of Walter Reed at the turn of the century (Bean, 1974, 1977). Reed's patient care guidelines were among the first to include procedures (such as informed consent) that are standard practice today. His consent forms included information on the experimental nature of treatments, were printed in both English and Spanish, and required the patient's written consent as well as Reed's signature as investigator (National Library of Medicine, 1986b). Writers of the history of medicine (Bean, 1974; 1977; DeKruf, 1926) give much evidence of Reed's lifelong commitment to ethics, humane care, and protecting patients' rights.

Ethical interventions such as Reed's were overshadowed in the twentieth century by unethical experiments that occurred in times of war and peace. Widespread governmental concern over involvement of humans in research arose following the abuse of large numbers of people in biomedical research during World War II. Experiments that humans were subjected to against their will included exposure to torturous extremes of temperature and altitude. As discussed previously, the *Nuremberg Code* established a precedent that exists today (National Library of Medicine, 1986b). Although those standards have existed since the late 1940s, in the United States there have been examples of subjects' rights abuses since that time. In the 1950s, jury panels were wiretapped without jurors' knowledge, allegedly to study group behavior (NLM, 1986b). Radiation experiments beginning in the 1940s injected patients with plutonium in northeastern U.S. hospitals without their knowledge, supposedly to study plutonium's effects ("Patients' Names Revealed," 1993). The Tuskegee syphilis experiments documented by Jones (1993) allowed nearly 300 African American men to be unaware of their diagnosis and deprived of treatment for nearly forty years, to study the course of the disease. Psychologists conducted ethically questionable research as well—for example, the well-known Milgram "obedience to authority" experiment (1974), which would never have received IRB approval had current standards been applied at the time.

These events collectively created a national awareness of the *need* for improved rights for patients and research participants. On July 1, 1966, the U.S. Surgeon General mandated that all research conducted that used human subjects must first be evaluated by a review board (Levine, 1986). In the 1970s, Congress established the National Commission for the Protection of Human Subjects of Biomedical and Behavioral Research, and passed the National Research Act, the first law to require that all studies funded by the (then) Department of Health, Education and Welfare be reviewed for ethical compliance. The National Commission conferenced in Maryland at the Belmont Center and in 1978 issued the Belmont Report, a document that detailed all institutional review board practices commonly used today (NLM, 1986). There are an estimated 3000 or more IRBs nationwide and more than 500 in other countries.

IRB Roles, Responsibilities, and Criteria

An IRB exists primarily to safeguard the welfare of patients or participants who will be studied in a research project. An IRB is required to evaluate all proposals on the basis of identical criteria based on both general and specific principles. The Belmont Report provided a model for evaluating research on two primary levels, referred to in this chapter as the *three ethical principles* and the *six points of procedure*, respectively.

Three Ethical Principles

The National Commission that wrote the Belmont Report noted that the principles put forth in the 1978 report have been part of patient care since the time of Hippocrates. In striving to continue the use of such principles in the twentieth century, the Commission tried to relate each point to data and actual research examples that IRBs could use. The three overarching ethical principles IRBs must follow are (a) respect for persons and their capabilities, including the idea that those with diminished autonomy, such as minors, are entitled to protection; (b) beneficence, or the dedication to the fact that the investigator will not harm the research participant physically or psychologically, will minimize risk of harm, and maximize possible benefits; and (c) justice, or the idea that all individuals should be treated equally and fairly in research investigations (NLM, 1986c). The concept of respect for persons, furthermore, embodies at least two specific ethical convictions. The first is that individuals should be considered "autonomous agents," capable of thinking clearly about their personal goals (NLM, 1986c); and that research participants should be dealt with openly and fairly. Beneficence as an ethical principal allows participants to trust those who conduct research. The Hippocratic oath principle of "first do no harm" is at its core. Finally, justice as a guiding strategy implies careful scrutiny of any process by which research participants are selected. It answers questions such as which persons should receive the benefits of research, and which should bear the risks, and insists that those who are confined, such as the institutionalized, shall not be singled out because of convenience or availability (NLM, 1986c).

Six Points of Procedure

The three principles can be thought of as being operationalized or executed in practice via one or more elements of the research procedure an investigator would typically be asked to adhere to by an IRB. IRBs complying with Belmont Report regulations must always use at least six criteria in evaluating a proposal (NLM, 1986c). These six criteria, and their relationship to the previously mentioned three principles, are listed in Table 7-1.

The first item in Table 7-1, "use fully informed consent," operationalizes the principle of respect for persons. This criterion is considered the single most important criterion that ethical research must follow. *Fully informed voluntary consent* implies (a) that the consent practices employed by a researcher will give volunteers a complete explanation of all procedures (surveys, measurements, interventions) they will experience during the research; (b) that a consent will be made on the basis of volunteers' knowing about *all* possible benefits and risks, including the possibility for any amount or level of loss of time, comfort, or dignity; (c) that consent will include a statement of the participants' absolute right to withdraw from the research at any point in time, with no penalty to themselves or jeopardy to any previously prom-

Table 7-1

Evaluation Criteria IRBs Must Follow as Specified by OPRR and Ethical Principles Embodied by Each Criterion

Evaluation criterion	— embodies →	Ethical principle
Use fully informed consent		Respect for persons
Protect confidentiality and privacy		Respect for persons
Minimize risk in research wherever and whenever possible		Respect for persons
Specify only risks that are acceptable given expected benefits		Beneficence
Provide continuous monitoring of data		Beneficence
Use an equitable procedure for selecting participants		Justice

ised remuneration, treatment, or other benefits; and (d) an understanding that the responsibility for ensuring that the participant can understand consent procedures rests with the investigator. Finally, IRBs must ensure that when *written* consent is required (in the case of any experiment with measurable risk) that only IRB-approved forms are used by investigators. The next two items in Table 7-1, "protect confidentiality and privacy" and "minimize risk wherever possible," also relate to the principle of respect for persons. The second item signifies that an IRB must not approve any research unless there is certainty that no one will have access to the data collected, other than the investigators and as few other individuals (such as research assistants) who must know something about responses to assist in the research. This is particularly important in the case of projects in which release of information on participation could be damaging to a volunteer's social status or employment (e.g., AIDS vaccine trials, research on attitudes or behaviors regarding sensitive areas such as drug use or sexual practices). The third item, "minimize risk wherever and whenever possible," requires researchers to guarantee every possible precaution for keeping negative side effects at an absolute minimum.

The fourth item, "specify only risks that are acceptable given the expected benefits," operationalizes the ethical principle of beneficence. It implies that the protocol, or procedure, for research is justified both from the point of view of scientific practice and also the welfare of the participant. It implies that the research is "worth doing" and will yield actual benefits for human participants. The fifth item, "provide continuous monitoring of data," is also intended to promote a beneficent approach to research. This item necessitates the continuous observation of subjects' performance through checking data for the participants' benefit, even to the point of termination of an experiment if data show negative effects that cannot be outweighed by any benefits. Similarly, some data collection or intervention procedures may induce negative emotional consequences that are not justifiable regardless of their potential for answering a research question (Gordon, Sugarman, & Kass, 1998). Finally, the last item, "use an equitable procedure for selecting participants," operationalizes the ethical principle of justice and requires IRBs to reject proposals that do not select participants fairly or overselect from vulnerable populations. OPRR instructional materials published by the NIH and the National Library of Medicine (1986a, 1986b, 1986c) caution IRBs to refuse consent to research that unjustifiably or disproportionately draws volunteers from populations that are vulnerable (e.g., those with malignant diseases), disenfranchised (prisoners, children), or unable to reasonably refuse (elderly individuals, psychiatric patients, medical students, or those with language difficulties). In summary, in evaluating a proposal as ethical and scientific, an IRB will review all information necessary to ensure that the proposed experiment follows Belmont Report mandates for *informed consent; specification of risks and benefits;* and *selection of participants,* adhering to principles of respect for persons, beneficence, and justice. OPRR guidelines are explicit, furthermore, in specifying that IRB approval is not unconditional nor irrevocable (NLM, 1986c).

The IRB Review and Decision-Making Process

Level of Risk

The IRB process usually begins with the IRB chair, who will read a proposal and then make an initial decision about whether a project is a "risk" or "no-risk" project. Following that assessment, one of three things can occur with the proposal based on three levels of possible "risk."

The first possible outcome is that the project will be deemed a category I (risk-free) project. This is usually the case for anonymous, mailed surveys on innocuous topics, or anonymous, noninteractive observation of public behavior (e.g., shoppers at a mall). Alternatively, the project could be viewed a category II proposal, which is usually the decision for studies involving interviews or self-report measures or any data collected either one-on-one or in groups in which there is no psychological intervention or deception. In this case, several IRB members will be selected to review and evaluate the project's acceptability, and the approval will be conveyed to the investigator via a memo from the chair giving permission to begin. This level of review, also referred to as *expedited review*, is often the case for research on psychological topics that do not involve deception.

The third possible level of risk is category III, usually applied to studies involving invasive measurements (such as blood draws), interventions (such as those involving exercise and physical exertion by volunteers), asking about sensitive topics (e.g., sexuality, drug use), experiments involving deception, or use of "special" populations such as minors or prisoners. Category III proposals require the use of written informed consent forms. Also, approval of category III proposals requires a meeting of all of the members of the IRB before approval can be granted. Usually, investigator(s) are given the option of attending the meeting with the IRB so that any questions or concerns can be answered immediately.

Typical IRB Concerns

The most common questions or requests for clarification that an IRB will ask deal with the matter of informed consent. For example, IRB members may ask for more information or more detail on the written informed consent form when one is necessary. They may raise concerns about the experimental nature of a treatment not being adequately addressed in the consent or lack of clarity over whether the principal investigator is faculty or a student. IRB members will also confirm that the informed consent form clearly states that confidentiality of the participants' identity is guaranteed if participation is not anonymous.

Another issue that is commonly raised in judging appropriateness of an informed consent form is potential that the written consent may hold for conveying a true level of voluntary "informed" consent from participants. IRBs will check to see that the form is phrased in the everyday language of the potential respondents and not "peppered" with psychological jargon that could mislead someone into volunteering. Waggoner and Mayo (1995), in a survey of 71 written informed consent forms used at a midwestern university, found that potential participants frequently did *not* understand language contained in recruitment letters or consent forms. Examples of terms misunderstood by most respondents to the consent forms, according to Waggoner and Mayo, included the words *waive, efficacy,* and *placebo.* Similarly, Gillespie (1994) recalled the example of a parent who misunderstood the sentence "Your child will be given a *battery* of tests" to mean that an electric shock was to be given to a young child. Kent (1996) summarized the findings of a number of studies on "readability" of consent forms, and cited examples of projects as sensitive as clinical trials for cancer using consent forms patients did not understand.

Another important issue IRB members will want to check is assurance that there is no coercion in participant recruitment, even of a very subtle or unintentional nature. To this end, IRB members will carefully examine methods of payment or remuneration offered participants. The two most common forms of recompense offered participants in both behavioral and biomedical experiments are extra course credit and cash. In the former example, it is extremely common (most of us went through it) to be recruited for participation in psychology experiments while in large, first-year classes. For these students, even one point of "extra credit" may be very appealing, regardless of what kind of experimental participation is required to obtain it. Similarly, medical schools often receive grants that include money for "subject payments." The participants these investigators then recruit could also be undergraduate students for whom a typical "honorarium" of $300 for full participation may seem like a fortune. Tragically, an incident just such as this may have occurred at a northeastern medical center when a 19-year-old sophomore died following a bronchoscopy conducted as part of university research that promised college volunteers a $150 payment for participation (Patrick, 1996). Many university psychology departments make the decision to *require* participation in experiments for all psychology students. They may do so to avoid this potential difficulty (i.e., the "enticement" of extra credit) and to guarantee availability of a participant pool. If this is communicated from the start, it may actually help students to identify with the research process and view it as a normal and expected responsibility and as their contribution to the scientific process.

IRB members may also have questions when there is use of deception in an experiment. If a project uses any kind of deception, the investigator must have a debriefing statement prepared that is shared with participants, explaining what the deception consisted of and clarifying any mistaken impressions the person may have gotten from not knowing this initially. Finally, if the research is not anonymous, and the participants will have to give their names, the researcher will have to explain the plan for safeguarding their identities (which can usually be accomplished by use of code numbers and storing consent forms and data separately).

Finally, faculty who wish to be as sensitive as possible to students' rights to informed consent should note that some IRBs consider review and approval preferable even when professors hand out personality measures in class, have their students complete them, then learn to score the measures by analyzing their own responses. This is more likely to be viewed as necessary by a college IRB when the class demonstrations include measures that have a clinical use (e.g., the MMPI, the Beck Depression Inventory). In the most stringent scenario, IRB review also applies to graduate students' recruiting friends for intellectual testing to allow "practice" administration of tests for courses in psychological assessment; faculty members who teach these courses are encouraged to check with the IRB before beginning graduate seminars that require test practice.

Recommendations for Negotiating the IRB Review Process

General Considerations in Contacts With the IRB

The first thing one should do in initiating the IRB process is to obtain IRB guidelines from one's university. This is usually easily accomplished. Contacting the chair of the IRB, even volunteering to go over to his or her office to pick them to allow the researcher to review them with the chair and ask any questions at that time is an excellent way to begin. If the university's IRB coordinator or chair is a member of the university's professional staff, he or she will do his or her best to take the time to meet with a researcher. At many places the IRB chair is a faculty member who may be juggling the usual full plate of teaching, research, and service activities. At many research universities the IRB chair or associate chair may have a full-time appointment in that role alone (Levine, 1986). At still other colleges the chair is staff rather than faculty. This is not something easily admitted by this author, but at most universities it can be more difficult to reach IRB chairs that are faculty, especially during summers. SUNY Brockport designates as IRB chair someone who is a member of the professional staff, and publicizes the fact that it is the IRB chair's responsibility to address all concerns and requests from faculty who solicit IRB approval, including meeting with individual faculty (especially if a meeting before the entire board to present the proposal will be required). Optimally, the IRB chair should also be willing to read rough drafts of the research proposal and give feedback prior to the submission of the final draft.

Preparing the Proposal

The components of the written summary researchers will have to submit share commonalties at all universities. The *minimum* elements required in the proposal will include (a) a description, (b) the informed consent form planned for administration to participants, and (c) a copy of each measure, survey, or interview that you will be using. The first part, the "project description," should be brief but should contain a description of objectives of the study, the planned methods, and the procedure for accomplishing data collection. Descriptions of statistical manipulation of the data postcollection is not necessary as an IRB's charge is only to examine procedures before and during data collection to ensure that participants' safety is ensured. If data are to be collected in an elementary/high school setting, a letter of support from the principal or district superintendent will be needed before the IRB can grant final approval.

Once the proposal is ready a faculty member will need to obtain signatures on it from colleagues who are coinvestigators (if any), and from the department head or chair. At that point, all materials can be forwarded to the IRB.

Attending IRB Meetings

Many IRBs allow faculty attendance during the meeting to review a given proposal. It is the personal feeling of this author that attending the IRB meeting that will decide on your proposal is part of the ethical responsibility that researchers hold. If the option exists, by all means attend the IRB meetings. IRBs often contain representatives from some of a university's most prolific research departments. Talking with them may yield for one some helpful advice on research design, replicability, or countless other areas relevant to the research that IRB members become aware of in reviewing its ethical compliance. Also, attending an IRB meeting helps one feel more ownership in the process of getting one's research approved. It can also provide an excellent learning opportunity for your students if you are allowed to bring them with you. Finally, attending the meeting means receiving feedback more quickly. A faculty member should receive some idea from members at the time of the meeting that lets one know how soon members feel they can approve the project. Often, it will be the same day—the IRB chair will give the researcher a written approval form—at which time one is free to begin the research. There are four actual categories of response that IRBs can give (Levine, 1986): (a) *approved*, which means that the researcher may proceed immediately with no further elaboration of methods, and so forth, required; (b) *approved contingent on revisions*, which usually are specific in nature and result from problems the IRB has identified; (c) *tabled*, which usually occurs when there is insufficient information for the IRB to make a decision on the welfare of participants; and (d) *disapproved*. Levine (1986) noted that an IRB may choose to request that an investigator withdraw a proposal and rewrite it substantially rather than cancel the project entirely. In this light, rejections, cancellations, or abrupt terminations of faculty members' research can remain relatively infrequent.

Caveats for Faculty in the IRB Process

The first caveat that should likely be mentioned is that a researcher must not expect same-day turnaround on a proposal. Most IRB members are professors, and they *are* sympathetic to deadlines; to needing to get one's data collected before the end of the term; and other similar pressures. Nonetheless, they will still need to have 3 to 5 working days to read your proposal and schedule a meeting. Therefore, it is best not to wait until the latter part of a semester to begin projects that involve a semester-based calendar deadline. Another caution is that it is understandable, if a large subject pool is available, for a researcher to desire as much data as possible. In an exploratory study one may want to measure as many facets and nuances of behavior as possible. Here the scholar's viewpoint and the IRB strictures may conflict. It may be the view of the IRB that included in your study should be only those variables that clearly relate to the primary research question. IRB members may in some cases feel they have to disallow data that are not really germane to the research question.

IRBs are also likely to request changes in proposals that describe research with children or adolescents. Several issues in this area have been noted by writers of ethics (e.g., Phillips,

1994), and the most prominent involve questions of "consent" and the nature of topics being studied. "Passive consent"—or the practice of not assessing parental consent but only parental refusals—in including teenagers in survey research remains controversial and is often dealt with differently by different campus IRBs. Similarly, surveys with questions about behaviors that place adolescents at risk for disease, danger, or other of the "new morbidities" (violence, drugs, and early sexual activity) specified by Dryfoos (1994), remain questionable to many IRB members. In these cases, the beneficence principle and justifying the proposed risks is the faculty member's paramount task.

Being Proactive in the IRB Review Process

There are many actions a researcher can take to be well-informed of IRB procedures and to keep abreast of new developments in OPRR rules and regulations. Maintaining an active research program, regularly submitting proposals, and maintaining contact with one's IRB chair is one obvious way to ensure familiarity, but other steps can be taken in addition. Researchers must be familiar with the *Ethical Principles of the American Psychological Association* (APA, 1992), and all writers should also maintain familiarity with the sections on ethics that are contained in the APA's fourth edition of the *Publication Manual* (APA, 1994; see section 6.05 of the *Manual*).

Furthermore, reading the journal *IRB: A Review of Human Subjects Research* (published by the Hastings Center in Garrison, New York), is an effective way to learn of new developments in federal guidelines, read book reviews on the topic, and stay informed. *IRB* also presents an excellent publication outlet for faculty who conduct research on IRB issues. University libraries often carry *IRB* if their chair requests it, and, in addition, individual subscriptions are extremely reasonable ($44.00 per year). Finally, to truly experience all of an IRB's responsibilities, join one. Faculty members are often needed on the IRB, and becoming a member is often one of the most enjoyable "college service" assignments that a member of a psychology faculty can experience.

Benefits of Involvement in the IRB Process

Teaching and Mentoring

One becomes a better teacher of research methods by having proposals reviewed by an IRB. IRBs follow explicit guidelines that are easily broken down into concrete steps for graduate students and undergraduates alike. For the student, going through the process of having one's research proposal IRB-approved is something that students rarely encounter prior to beginning a master's thesis in graduate school, yet becoming familiar with the procedures as an undergraduate also carries with it many advantages. Formally submitting an IRB proposal, signed by one's faculty supervisor and department chair, helps identify the student as the primary investigator on the research and thus formalizes his or her ownership of the proposed project. Also, IRB contact familiarizes the student with federal guidelines for the protection of participants, a vital skill when they obtain faculty positions and undertake grant funding and major research projects of their own.

Gillespie and George (1998) surveyed a group of 33 undergraduate students who had proposals for research reviewed by an IRB. The authors used a self-report questionnaire that included Likert scale ratings of attitudes toward the IRB process; open-ended questions in which respondents could briefly describe their reactions and feelings to the IRB; and a brief adjective checklist. Adjectives on the checklist were eight positive feeling words (e.g., *helpful, enjoyable, educational*) and eight negative feeling words (e.g., *tedious, confusing, pointless*). Among their findings were that 60% of the students indicated that going through the IRB process had helped them with their career goals; 51% stated that they approach research in a different way after having learned about IRB procedures; and 69% rated the IRB review process as either *slightly helpful, moderately helpful,* or *very helpful* to them. Students were also asked if they would participate in the IRB review process again with a future project even if it were optional; 48% said yes, citing reasons that included "it helps you learn more about research," "it assures you your research is ethical," "it looks better if you publish your data," "it helps you articulate your research process," and "it helps you foresee problems with your research and correct them." Table 7-2 summarizes additional results.

Gillespie and George (1998) also noted that because federally funded mentoring programs now exist (the purpose of which are to encourage talented students to pursue graduate study), another avenue has opened for students to become well-acquainted with good research methods (including IRB review) during their undergraduate careers. One such program is the Ronald E. McNair Fellowship Program, named in honor of the African American astronaut who was among those killed in the shuttle *Challenger* explosion. At SUNY Brockport, all McNair Fellows (15 to 25 per year) must have their research reviewed by the IRB. In summary, the IRB process, far from being obstructionistic, can be an informative and enriching part of research mentoring.

Scholarship

The benefits of IRB contact for one's scholarship may be indirect. Not all IRB members publish frequently or conduct large research projects. However, all IRBs must require follow-up reports on an annual basis, for which the IRB chair will send memos to faculty requesting updates on the data collections for which they requested IRB approval. In short, regular contact with an IRB helps "keep one on one's toes" in meeting deadlines for completion of research, which ultimately strengthens scholarship efforts. In the case of a previous IRB review for a grant-funded project, regular IRB review virtually guarantees better scholarship, as grant renewals hinge on attaining excellence in results and method.

Service

The greatest guarantor that one will make a contribution in the area of service is simply by caring enough to be a member of an IRB. Universities regularly need new IRB members, in-

Table 7-2

Student Characteristics and Reactions to Participation in the IRB Review Process

	N	Percentage
Reason for research		
Class project	25/33	76
Independent study	5/33	15
McNair fellow	3/33	9
Topic of research		
Psychological	13/33	39
Health behavior-related	4/33	12
Physical education/sport	7/33	21
Other	9/33	27
Ratings of IRB process		
Perceived IRB helpfulness		
1 = not at all helpful	3/33	9
2 = neither helped nor hindered	7/33	21
3 = slightly helpful	7/33	21
4 = helpful	10/33	30
5 = very helpful	6/33	18
Perceived difficulty of IRB process		
1 = very difficult	0/33	0
2 = somewhat difficult	6/33	18
3 = neither difficult nor convenient	3/33	9
4 = reasonably convenient	15/33	45
5 = very convenient	9/33	27
Would request IRB review even if optional		
Yes	16/33	48
No	10/33	30
Not sure	7/33	21
Reasons would request IRB review even if optional		
Helps you learn more about research	3/16	19
Ensures that research is ethical	8/16	50
Looks better if you publish	1/16	6
Helps you articulate your methods	2/16	13
Helps you foresee problems with the research project	2/16	13

NOTE: 33 students responded to the survey; 16 indicated that they would request IRB review even if it were optional.

cluding faculty who passionately care about good science and research endeavors of the highest ethical standards. College service on an IRB may count significantly for younger faculty members seeking reappointment or tenure, although experts caution that IRB members should not hold any vested interests ("Researchers Face Likely Changes," 1998).

Ethics

It is ironic that IRBs, which should be at the leading edge of knowledge of ethics, have recently come under fire for not keeping up with changes in human subject research in the 1990s ("Researchers Face Likely Changes," 1998). Recent directives from the Office of the Inspector General of Health and Human Services (DHHS) recommend holding IRBs accountable for results of research, requiring IRBs to improve ways to protect human subjects at the actual research sites, require more diverse IRB membership, and require initial orientation and continuing education in ethics for members of IRBs. These changes can only make the IRB process better. In the long run, IRB contact will always improve one's knowledge of research ethics. At a time when applied research is delving into new and more controversial areas daily, and decisions on issues such as passive consent seem subject to political pressures ("Survey Research on Minors Is Safe, for Now," 1993), knowledge of the roles and history of IRBs provides some eternal truths to be relied on.

Conclusion

The interaction with IRBs that faculty members can incorporate into their daily work can be positive and rewarding. When faculty commit to work with their IRB as a colleague and an equal, and maintain a willingness and enthusiasm to learn the most that they can from the entire experience, it can be a partnership that benefits participants, IRB members, and researchers.

References

American Psychological Association. (1992). Ethical principles of psychologists and code of conduct. *American Psychologist, 47,* 1597–1611.

American Psychological Association. (1994). *Publication manual of the American Psychological Association* (4th ed.). Washington, DC: Author.

Bean, W. B. (1974). Walter Reed: A biographical sketch. *Archives of Internal Medicine, 134,* 871–877.

Bean, W. B. (1977). Walter Reed and the ordeal of human experiments. *Bulletin of the History of Medicine, 51,* 75–92.

DeKruf, P. (1926). Walter Reed: In the interest of science—and for humanity. In P. DeKruf (Ed.), *Microbe hunters* (pp. 311–333). San Francisco: Jossey-Bass.

Dryfoos, J. (1994). *Full-service schools: A revolution in mental health and social services for children, youth, and families.* San Francisco: Jossey-Bass.

Gillespie, J. F. (1994). *The ten steps of a good assessment process.* Unpublished manuscript.

Gillespie, J. F., & George, K. (1998, March). *Institutional review boards and training in research: Students' reactions to the process.* Paper presented in the 15th Annual Scholars' Day Symposium at SUNY College at Brockport, Brockport, NY.

Gordon, V. M., Sugarman, J., & Kass, N. (1998). Toward a more comprehensive approach to protecting human subjects. *IRB: A Review of Human Subjects Research, 20,* 1–5.

Jones, J. H. (1993). *Bad blood: The Tuskegee syphilis experiment.* New York: Free Press.

Kent, G. (1996). Shared understandings for informed consent: The relevance of psychological research on the provision of information. *Social Science and Medicine, 43,* 1517–1523.

Levine, R. J. (1986). The institutional review board. In *Ethics and regulation of clinical research* (2nd ed.). Baltimore: Urban & Schwartzberg.

Milgram, S. L. (1974). *Obedience to authority: An experimental view.* New York: Harper & Row.

National Library of Medicine (Producer), & Slatkin, C. (Editor). (1986a). *Evolving concerns in ethics.* [Videocassette] (Available from the National Library of Medicine, Bethesda, MD)

National Library of Medicine (Producer), & Slatkin, C. (Editor). (1986b). *The Belmont Report: Basic ethical principles and their applications* [Videocassette] (Available from the National Library of Medicine, Bethesda, MD)

National Library of Medicine (Producer), & Slatkin, C. (Editor). (1986c). *Balancing society's mandate: IRB Review Criteria.* [Videocassette] (Available from the National Library of Medicine, Bethesda, MD)

Patients' names revealed. (1993, November 16). *Democrat & Chronicle* (Rochester, NY), 1A, 6A.

Patrick, K. (1996, April 14). Students, others at UR grieve for friend. *Times-Union* (Rochester, NY), 1B.

Phillips, S. R. (1994). Asking the sensitive question: The ethics of survey research and teen sex. *IRB: A Review of Human Subjects Research, 16,* 1–7.

Researchers face likely changes as ethics boards come under scrutiny. (1998, June). *Federal Grants & Contracts Weekly, 22,* 1, 12.

Rosnow, R. L., Rotheram-Borus, M. J., Ceci, S. J., Blanck, P. D., & Koocher, G. P. (1993). The institutional review board as a mirror of scientific and ethical standards. *American Psychologist, 48,* 821–826.

Survey research on minors is safe, for now. (1996, November). *APS Observer,* 3.

Waggoner, W. C., & Mayo, D. M. (1995). Who understands? A survey of 25 words or phrases commonly used in proposed clinical research consent forms. *IRB: A Review of Human Subjects Research, 17,* 6–9.

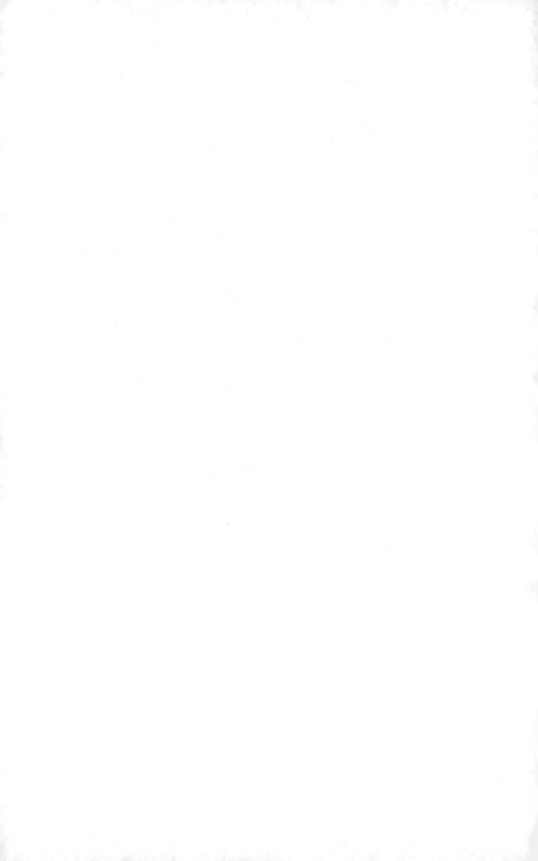

IV

Vulnerable Populations
and Risks of Research

This final section describes specific problems attendant to conducting research with special populations that may be more vulnerable to research risk and research on controversial topics.

Chapter 8 is a report of the results of a survey of the interactions between IRBs and researchers studying controversial topics. Included are issues such as factors that IRBs weigh most heavily, the impact of research funding on IRB approval, and the topics, populations, and procedures that are considered to be controversial by IRBs. Ways to reduce friction between these parties are suggested.

Chapter 9 provides information regarding the concerns of IRBs and researchers when DPSs are involved in human sexuality research. Similarities and differences in the views of these groups are outlined, and the complex issues that arise are discussed.

Interactions Concerning Risky Research: Investigators Rate Their IRBs (and Vice Versa)

James R. Council, Elizabeth J. H. Smith,
Jessica Kaster-Bundgaard,
and Brian A. Gladue

Psychologists conducting human research can hardly escape dealing with an Institutional Review Board (IRB). Although a number of mechanisms exist in this country to protect research participants, the IRB is paramount in most organizations. IRBs have been created at research institutions to ensure the ethical treatment of research participants (OPRR, 1991). They exist in all organizations that receive federal funding for human subject research and most colleges and universities require that nonfunded research be reviewed under the same guidelines. These committees have members of varying backgrounds, including nonprofessionals, to ensure that the academic and larger communities are fully represented.

In an ideal situation, researchers should welcome input from IRBs to ensure that every possible step is taken to pro-

Portions of this research were presented at the Midwestern Psychological Conference, May 1996, Chicago; at the conference of the Society of Clinical and Experimental Hypnosis, November 1995, San Antonio, TX; and in the *American Journal of Clinical Hypnosis* (Council et al., 1997).

tect their participants from undue risk. In reality, relations between researchers and IRBs may become strained as a result of conflicting perceptions, motivations, and goals. The researcher would like to gain information about some aspect of human functioning as quickly, efficiently, and validly as possible. Opposed to this is the IRB's responsibility to protect the welfare of the research participants. Strictly speaking, the IRB is not particularly interested in the knowledge the researcher hopes to gain. The theoretical or social importance of a study only comes into consideration when it is necessary to justify procedures involving more than minimal risk.

IRB members seem to feel misunderstood and unappreciated by researchers, and vice versa. Although researchers complain about red tape and misplaced priorities, IRBs cannot understand researchers' failure to appreciate the importance of ethical safeguards (Gilbert, 1983; Murray, 1984). Furthermore, the openness about purposes and procedures demanded by IRBs may be antithetical to the researcher's desire to minimize demand effects and other biasing influences. For example, informed consent is central to ethical research practices (Kimmel, 1979; Sieber, 1993; Stanley, Sieber, & Melton, 1987), but fully informing participants about experimental procedures could jeopardize the validity of many psychology studies. Some researchers justify the active deception of participants to disguise more completely the purpose of an experiment. However, because of ethical constraints, deception is not nearly as common in psychological research as it once was. To use deception, investigators must now provide "elaborate justifications and extensive debriefing procedures" (Kimmel, 1979, p. 643). Not only IRB guidelines, but also the APA's principles of research ethics hold that deceptive practices should be employed only if absolutely necessary (APA, 1992; see page 13, standard 6.15).

We may be exaggerating the polarization between IRBs and researchers, but when researchers or IRB members talk among themselves the antagonism toward the "other side" is often readily apparent. Because two of the authors of this chapter (Council and Gladue) have sat on and chaired university IRBs, as well as conducted extensive research in areas considered to entail more than minimal risk, we were aware of the issues from both perspectives. As researchers on hypnosis and human sexuality, most of the comments about IRBs we heard from colleagues were negative. However, our own experiences indicated that IRBs were sympathetic to investigators and approached their task of protecting the rights of research subjects constructively. Were our IRB experiences atypical, or were we just hearing the complaints of a vocal minority of investigators? These questions provided the starting point for a survey investigating the interactions of researchers and IRBs. We believed that it would be important to examine the IRB process both from the perspective of the researcher and the IRB. Our questions for researchers addressed issues such as the following: To which factors do IRBs give the greatest attention? Do IRBs understand the nature and methodology of your research area? Is the review process constructive and efficient? Does the population from which research participants are drawn make a difference? Does serving on an IRB affect your perceptions of the review process? Does it matter if your research is funded or not? If there was one thing you could change about your IRB, what would it be?

Our questions for IRBs complemented those we had for researchers: What kinds of research topics, populations, and procedures do IRBs view as being particularly risky? What can researchers do to facilitate the review process? If there was one thing you could change about your IRB, what would it be? In addition, we examined IRB composition and procedures.

Plan of the Study

Our original purpose was to examine the IRB process with regard to hypnosis and sex research, our own special interests. Although a brief report for hypnosis researchers has already been published (Council, Smith, Bundgaard, & Gladue, 1997), there was much additional information of general interest in our findings. For one thing, space constraints prevented Council et al. (1997) from quoting responses to open-ended questions. Several other factors justified a reanalysis of the data for the current volume. First, our survey instruments were disguised to avoid revealing our specific interest in hypnosis and sex research, and many respondents indicated that their primary research interests were in other areas. We used these surveys to form an "other" group for comparison with the hypnosis and sex researchers, and our analyses revealed virtually no mean differences between the groups on survey responses (Council et al., 1997). Thus we felt comfortable combining our researcher groups into a single sample.

Our methodology followed Dillman's (1978) recommendations. We mailed surveys to 137 researchers belonging to hypnosis societies, and 166 researchers belonging to organizations concerned with human sexuality. Follow-up reminders were sent to participants who had not returned their surveys after 2 months, and the final sample included responses from 176 investigators. To conform to this volume's emphasis on IRBs and departmental subject pools, we have limited our present analyses to 116 researchers who indicated that they primarily used college students in their studies.

Included in materials sent to researchers was a parallel survey to be forwarded to their institution's IRB. If we received a completed survey from an investigator but did not receive a corresponding IRB survey, we called the institution, located the appropriate administrator, and sent that person a survey. A total of 76 IRB administrators returned completed surveys. For both investigators and IRBs, the surveys consisted of objective and free-response items. Free-response items were independently scored by two raters, and proportion agreement ranged from .82 to .96.

Results and Discussion

Survey of Investigators

Our sample consisted primarily of investigators engaged in research on sex (38%) or hypnosis (30%). Other areas of research included emotions (5%), psychotherapy (5%), abuse (2%), drugs (2%), or "other" areas (18%)—for example, exercise, sleep loss, and pain. Most investigators (65%) reported that they had submitted fewer than five projects to their IRBs during the past 3 years. Seventy-seven percent reported that none of their projects had been reviewed under the exempt category. Exempt projects (e.g., anonymous surveys) are low-risk and approved administratively without going through committee. On average, only one of our respondents' projects received an expedited review, which can be done through correspondence. In contrast, an average of 2.4 research projects received a full board review, which is the highest level of scrutiny, and entails a personal meeting of the investigator and committee. We were successful, therefore, in contacting a sample engaged in research involving more than minimal risk.

Our list of risky research topics included sexual behavior, hypnosis, drugs, aggression, emotions, psychotherapy, trauma, abuse, and other. Of these topics, 47% of investigators reported that they had submitted a project concerned with sexual behavior to their IRBs, and 39% had submitted a hypnosis project. Investigators had also submitted research projects concerned with emotions (25%), psychotherapy (18%), drugs (14%), aggression (6%), trauma (3%), and abuse (12%). Examples of protocols submitted under the other category (33%) included projects on sleep loss, exercise, and pain control. (Respondents could endorse more than one category.)

Investigators were also asked to rate the level of scrutiny of their projects by their IRBs on a scale of 1 (*no attention*) to 5 (*painstaking examination*). The majority of researchers reported that the IRB gave moderate or no attention to factors such as the merit of the project ($M = 2.27$), scientific basis for the project ($M = 2.51$), benefits to the subjects or to society ($M = 2.33$; $M = 2.78$), and compensation to the subjects ($M = 2.19$). However, investigators believed that the IRB gave considerably more attention to the subjects' welfare ($M = 4.04$), risks to the subjects ($M = 4.20$), and the wording of the consent form ($M = 4.22$). These results indicate that

IRBs tend to conform to the emphases indicated in the OPRR (1991) guidelines for the protection of human subjects.

When asked whether the IRB understood the nature of their research, 47% of the investigators said that the IRB did not understand the nature of their research, compared to 53% who said their IRB did understand. Most investigators (53%) reported that the IRB understood commonly accepted practices and procedures associated with their research, although 41% believed the IRB did not. Fifty-four percent of the investigators reported that they had tried to educate their IRB with regard to their research area. The ways in which researchers attempted to educate their IRB included "overly [explaining] procedures in proposals"; "citing literature concerning low risk"; and "providing extensive background in writing each time we submit [a protocol]." Investigators' ratings of IRB criticism of various factors in research protocols indicate IRBs had very few problems or objections regarding factors such as the validity of their methodology, scientific merit, social benefits, and personal benefits to subjects. Although investigators rated *risk to subject* as drawing more criticism than the other factors, the mean for this category indicated only very minor objections. In rating how IRBs handled their projects, investigators tended to describe IRBs as timely and efficient, although they were less positive with respect to the IRB's understanding of experimental procedures, background principles, and constructive criticism. Because some of our investigators reported using both college student and other populations in their research, we examined whether using populations other than college students increased IRB estimates of risk. Only 7% said their IRB perceived their research as *less* risky if they used populations other than college students, whereas 32% reported that using populations other than college students (i.e., psychiatric patients, medical patients, children) increased the IRB's estimate of risk associated with their research. As one investigator said, "It's one reason why I use students and not patients."

When asked to compare their experiences with their IRBs to those of colleagues working on similar research at other institutions, 30% of investigators reported that their experiences were better than those of their colleagues and 32% stated their experiences were the same, whereas only 8% reported that their experiences were worse than those of their colleagues. However, 28% of the investigators stated that their experiences with their IRBs were worse than those of colleagues working in different areas of research at their institution. Only 14% reported that their experiences were better compared with other researchers at their institution. The majority of researchers (66%) were either very or somewhat satisfied with past IRB experiences, whereas 19% were very or somewhat dissatisfied with their past IRB experiences.

Researchers were divided about whether a research project's funding status influenced IRB decisions. Thirty-eight percent reported that funding might bear on an IRB's decisions, compared with 39% who felt that funding did not have any bearing on IRB decisions.

When asked, "If there was any one thing you could change about your IRB, what would it be?" 32% indicated that they would like to change the procedures, process, and paperwork involved; 38% wanted to change the IRB's understanding of different types of research; 8% wanted to get rid of the IRB entirely; and 17% indicated that they did not want to change anything.

Sixty-eight percent of our investigators had served on their institution's IRB, and of these, 84% had served as chair. We attempted to determine the effects of serving on an IRB by conducting t tests on responses to appropriate items. For the majority of items, investigators who had served on their institution's IRB responded similarly to investigators who had not served on their institution's IRB. However, those who had served on an IRB indicated that the IRB gave *more attention* to a project's benefit to society (t [102] = 2.46, p = .01), and *less criticism* concerning risks to participants (t [108] = −2.25, p < .05) than those who had not served. Investigators who had served on IRBs characterized them as being *more efficient* in handling projects (t [114] = 2.00, p < .05), giving *more constructive criticism* (t [110] = 2.15, p < .05), being *better informed* (t [110] = 2.36, p < .01), and having a *better understanding* of experimental procedures (t [110] 2.10, p < .05). Furthermore, investigators who had *not* served were more dissatisfied with their past IRB experiences than were investigators who had served (t [108] = -2.60, $p < .01$).

Survey of IRB Administrators

Results of the survey (see Table 8-1) indicated that typically, about 75% of a university's IRB is comprised of male mem-

Table 8-1

Composition of IRBs

Category	All (100%)	Mostly (75%)	Half (50%)	Some (25%)	None (0%)
Gender:					
Male	0	61	35	4	0
Female	0	4	35	61	0
Age:					
25–45	0	25	48	25	1
45–65	1	24	49	23	3
Academics					
Active researchers					
Human research	5	34	33	28	0
Animal research	0	4	1	53	42
Nonresearch academics	1	7	9	54	0
Administrators	0	0	1	73	25
Laypersons:					
Attorneys	0	0	0	63	37
Clergy	0	0	0	55	45
Other	0	0	4	65	32

NOTE: Numbers in the table refer to the percentage of IRB administrators endorsing a certain category of composition. For example, 35% of the respondents indicated that their IRBs were made up of 50% male and 50% female members. Percentages attached to categories are approximate; for example, "some (25%)" should be taken to indicate the presence of one or more of a type of representative.

bers; 25% of IRB members are doing animal research; and approximately 50% are engaged in human research. Survey results also suggest that fewer than one quarter of an institution's IRB is composed of nonresearch academics or laypersons. Attorneys are often included on IRBs and are actively involved in the decision-making process. Most IRB administrators (58%) indicated that the attorney was affiliated with their institution. Results showed that most IRBs meet on a bimonthly (24%) or monthly (52%) basis. The mean number of protocols submitted per year to the IRB for any kind of review was 283, and 21% of those protocols required major revisions before being approved.

Although some large research universities permit reviews by departmental IRBs, 94% of the IRB administrators in our sample indicated that a central IRB reviewed all research conducted in their institution. The most frequently evaluated protocols were in the areas of clinical trials of drug effects (20%) and in survey research on emotions (10%). These characteristics correspond closely to those found in a national survey of university IRBs by Hayes, Hayes, and Dykstra (1995).

Perception of Risk

IRB administrators were asked to rate how much risk was associated with various research topics (i.e., sexual behavior, hypnosis, drugs, emotions). Although mean IRB responses (see Figure 8-1) indicate that these research areas entailed at least minimal risk, it appears that survey research was seen as posing less risk than experimental manipulations or laboratory studies. Free-response data suggested other research considered very risky included topics related to HIV and AIDS, strenuous physical activity, alcohol use, depression, and manipulation of emotions.

We also addressed research involving deception, asking whether there were any particular combinations (e.g., deception in drug trials) which raised red flags with the committee. Almost half of the respondents answered that *any* deception raises red flags. Typical comments included, "Deception is

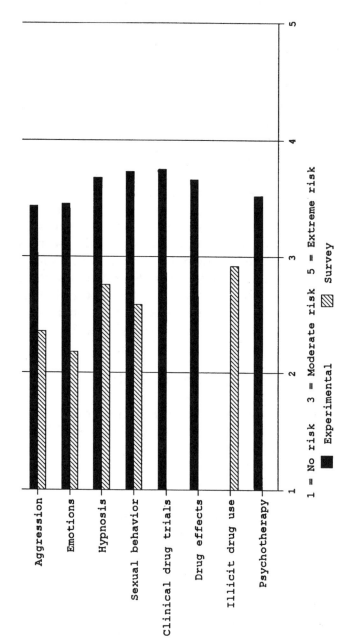

Figure 8-1. IRB administrators' ratings of research risks.

always a red flag. The committee considers the use of deception seriously in relation to the necessity for its use and its
potential threat," and "We recently refused to approve two
protocols because the ends did not justify the means." Comments on combinations of factors that raise red flags included
the following: "Misinforming participants about potential
effects–risks in drug studies"; "placebo in drug trials"; "Deception with children and elderly or minority populations is
a major red flag for us"; "deception in administering alcohol"; "deception in depression and anxiety studies; deception
with studies involving children"; "deception with drug effects"; "Deception regarding legal limits of confidentiality, although in many cases this is probably unintentional"; "deception in informed consent"; "deception with children or
mentally–emotionally disabled persons."

We also investigated whether the level of risk might vary
with the population being studied by asking respondents to
indicate whether various topics were particularly risky for
various populations. Chi-square analyses indicated that the
level of risk for research areas such as sex (χ^2 [6, n = 294] =
33.57, p < .001), hypnosis (χ^2 [6, n = 274] = 15.55, p < .01),
aggression (χ^2 [6, n = 271] = 23.64, p < .001), emotions (χ^2 [6,
n = 262] = 20.24, p < .01), and psychotherapy (χ^2 [6, n = 262]
= 16.50, p < .01), varies depending on the population under
study. (See Table 8-2.) For example, sex research with children
under 12, adolescents, and mentally retarded persons was
more often cited as risky than sex research with college students, medical patients, or prisoners. It is interesting to note
that drug research was viewed as equally risky for college
students, medical patients, psychiatric patients, children and
adolescents, prisoners, and mentally retarded participants.
Comments with regard to this question included the following: "Level of risk is judged less by the topic than by the
particular research procedures used. Areas of concern are
confidentiality, psycho-social risk and risk of physical injury"; "All [topics] could be 'risky' under certain circumstances"; "All of the topics could be risky with all of
the defined groups—depending on the methods used, etc.";
"It really depends on whether the research is 'invasive' in

Table 8-2

Percentages of IRB Administrators Endorsing a Research Topic as Risky for a Special Population (in percentages)

Research topic	Population						
	College students	Medical patients	Psychiatric patients	Children under 12	Children over 12	Prisoners	Mentally retarded individuals
Sex	37	26	49	78	76	50	71
Hypnosis	37	34	50	66	65	46	63
Drugs	61	65	59	76	78	63	71
Aggression	34	28	60	67	59	59	68
Emotions	34	28	54	61	59	42	67
Psychotherapy	36	32	47	65	58	49	63

the sense of experimental manipulation being used vs. survey/correlational. All of these would be considered risky if they were 'invasive.'"

In constructing the survey, we thought it would be important to give IRB administrators an opportunity to air their "pet peeves." Making researchers more aware of such problems could greatly facilitate their relations with IRBs. Table 8-3 summarizes the responses to this item. Overwhelmingly, administrators ranked "problems with consent forms and related documents" as the major problem in dealing with researchers. (Typically, IRBs request that researchers follow a standard format for submitting their protocols; quite often investigators fail to follow the guidelines.) Other pet peeves included the following: "Poorly conceived protocols"; "Using self as the IRB 'expert' "; "Use of classroom time to accomplish research unrelated to the class (problem of captive population)"; "Faculty members who decide on their own that they do not need human subjects clearance"; "Changes in consent form and other material after committee review process which changes consent forms acceptability to the committee."

Given the opportunity to change one thing about the IRB at their institution, 30% of administrators said they would

Table 8-3

Percentage of Administrators Ranking Problem as "Most Important"

Problem	Percentage
Consent forms and related documents	65
Misunderstanding IRB regulations	10
Investigator failure to meet IRB deadlines	9
Incomplete forms	7
Timeliness of annual updates	5
Other (conducting research without submitting protocol for review; research on students without IRB knowledge; lack of institutional recognition and support)	4

change factors such as procedures, paperwork, speed of review, or the general IRB process; 28% would like to change issues surrounding education and understanding of different types of research; and 15% indicated that they would not change anything.

Conclusion

Our findings can be summarized to indicate that investigators who conduct research involving more than minimal risk with department subject pools are fairly well-satisfied with their IRBs. According to the investigators, IRBs tend to conform to their mission of safeguarding the rights of research participants. Problems with approval of a research protocol are much more likely to stem from IRB concerns about the welfare or rights of participants than from criticisms of the scientific merit or social benefits of the project. However, a substantial proportion of investigators did not feel that IRBs really understood the nature of their research. Many of the investigators in our sample had actually served on their IRBs, and this exposure seemed to lead to better understanding and more positive perceptions of IRB procedures.

For their part, IRBs seem to give appropriate attention to projects relative to the topics, methods, and populations involved. The use of deception gives IRBs particular concern. Investigators would be well advised to use only the level of deception necessary to achieve the aims of a project, as well as to provide thorough justification for any deceptive procedures. Finally, it should be of some comfort to researchers to find that IRBs agree with them that the amount of time and paperwork involved in the review process is a problem.

We will end by using our personal experiences to expand on our findings and suggest ways to facilitate IRB–investigator interactions. The main findings are congruent with our own observations as investigators, IRB members, and IRB chairs. Although serious in their mission, IRBs are sympathetic to researchers and strive to be constructive rather than obstructive. This is probably the main reason why the investigators in our sample were basically satisfied with their IRBs. The fact that IRBs perceive college students as less vulnerable than other populations undoubtedly contributes to positive interactions between IRBs and investigators who use departmental subject pools.

Despite our generally encouraging findings, responses on both sides indicated that researchers and IRBs in some institutions had fallen into adversarial relationships. Because of an IRB's ability to veto or significantly alter a research project, investigators may be primed to perceive abuses of power. We believe that by virtue of their having the upper hand, IRBs should take the initiative in facilitating positive and constructive interactions. The pains an IRB takes to promote a positive image and relationships are minor compared to those stemming from investigators viewing it as "the enemy."

In our experience, *education, facilitation,* and *flexibility* are essential for IRBs to maintain positive and effective interactions with researchers. IRBs should *educate* investigators not only about rules and regulations but in the principles, rationale, and history of protecting human subjects. When investigators express annoyance with IRBs, it is often because they view their own research as innocuous and cannot see the need for oversight. Clinical investigators who pursue overtly risky topics seem most accepting of regulation, because in those cases the need is so clear. Education can help all investigators understand how ethical principles apply to them. In an ideal situation, this process should start at the undergraduate level and should receive significant attention during graduate school. IRBs can promote education by sending representatives to classes and faculty meetings, and making materials on research ethics available to instructors.

By *facilitation* we mean that IRBs should make the process of gaining approval for a research protocol as easy and painless as possible. IRBs should strive to be open and accommodating to researchers. At North Dakota State University, the IRB maintains a Web site, publishes a column in a university newsletter, and tries to keep paperwork straightforward and understandable. Most important, the IRB staff are accessible and responsive, so that questions are answered and paperwork processed quickly. Taking time at the beginning to guide new investigators through the process pays off in the long run.

Finally, *flexibility* is essential to combat the image of the IRB as a hidebound bureaucracy. Investigators may have research opportunities come up unexpectedly, graduate students facing deadlines, practical constraints, or other situations requiring a relaxation of usual IRB procedures. IRBs have considerable latitude in many situations, and we have found that accommodating researchers' special needs pays great dividends in future good will.

On the researchers' part, an appreciation of the constraints and pressures under which IRBs operate should promote some sympathy and appreciation. Although IRBs are intended to be grassroots organizations with considerable autonomy, they must still follow a complex set of federal and university guidelines. Furthermore, the tasks of IRBs are often complicated by the necessity of functioning with minimal resources. Investigators who understand this and facilitate the IRB process by mastering the rules and paperwork are likely to have better experiences with their IRBs. Being aware of which procedures raise red flags (e.g., deception) can also be helpful.

Investigators should also use education to facilitate their interactions with IRBs. On one hand, this can take the form of educating IRBs about one's research area—for example, by providing documentation or background on one's procedures. On the other hand, researchers can educate themselves about the review process by serving on their IRBs. Overall, our results suggest that the more researchers and IRBs know about each other's domains, the more productive their interactions will be.

References

American Psychological Association Ethics Committee. (1992). Ethical principles of psychologists and code of conduct. *American Psychologist, 47*, 1597–1611.

Council, J. R., Smith, E. J. H., Bundgaard, J., & Gladue, B. (1997). Ethical evaluation of hypnosis research: A survey of investigators and their institutional review boards. *American Journal of Clinical Hypnosis, 39*, 258–265.

Dillman, D. A. (1978). *Mail and telephone surveys: The total design method.* New York: J. Wiley & Sons.

Gilbert, S. J. (1983). The behavior of non-psychologists on review committees. *American Psychologist, 38*, 123–125.

Hayes, G. J., Hayes, S. C., & Dykstra, T. (1995). A survey of university Institutional Review Boards: Characteristics, policies, and procedures. *IRB: A Review of Human Subjects Research, 17*, 1–6.

Kimmel, A. J. (1979). Ethics and human subjects research: A delicate balance. *American Psychologist, 34*, 633–635.

Murray, T. H. (1984). Comment on Gilbert. *American Psychologist, 39*, 812–813.

Office for Protection from Research Risks. (1991). *Protection of human subjects* (DHHS publication No. 99-158). Washington, DC: U.S. Government Printing Office.

Sieber, J. E. (1993). Ethical considerations in planning and conducting research on human subjects. *Academic Medicine, 68*, s9–s13.

Stanley, B., Sieber, J. E., & Melton, G. B. (1987). Empirical studies of ethical issues in research. *American Psychologist, 42*, 735–741.

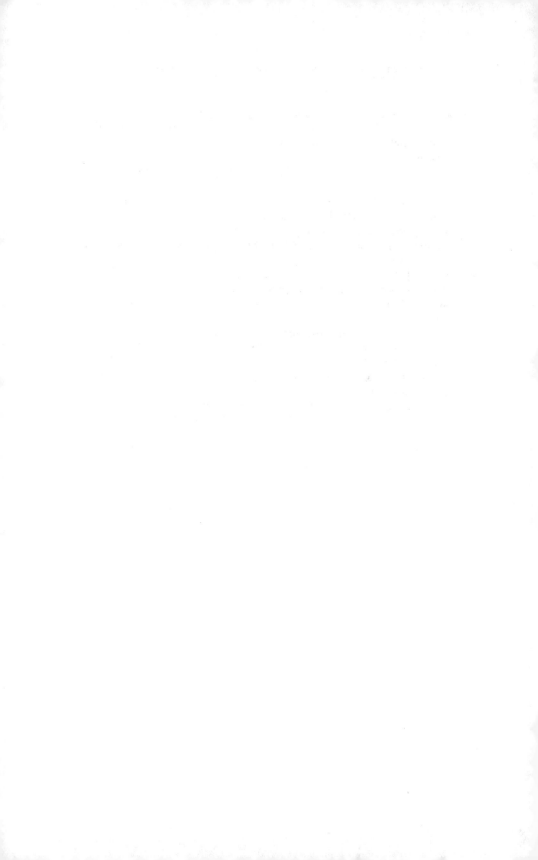

Chapter

9

Sexuality Research, Institutional Review Boards, and Subject Pools

Michael W. Wiederman

Because of its private nature, human sexuality research typically involves self-report of experience, behavior, and attitudes. To investigate most psychological and behavioral facets of human sexuality, researchers must rely on self-report data of some form. Although it is true that some researchers attempt to directly measure physiological response to sexual stimuli, perusal of journals in which sexuality research is published quickly reveals the heavy reliance on self-report. In the typical sexuality study in the behavioral sciences, respondents are presented with direct questions or previously published surveys. These latter items frequently consist of a series of statements toward which the respondent indicates his or her degree of agreement using a Likert-type scale. Although such studies can be conducted using face-to-face interviews, self-administered questionnaires are the norm.

Human sexuality research also is heavily dependent on college student participants. Carri Maynard, Carrie Fretz, and I conducted a content analysis of every research article published between 1970 and 1995 in the leading human sexuality research journals, *The Journal of Sex Research* and *Archives of Sexual Behavior*. I will allude to some of the findings of this analysis later in this chapter. At this point, however, it is important to note that one half of the samples used in these articles were made up of college students. Accordingly, issues involving sexuality research, student subject pools, and IRB concerns are relevant to each other.

The purpose of this chapter is to highlight some of the primary concerns raised by IRBs and researchers when sexuality research is conducted with participants drawn from departmental subject pools. In so doing, I hope to accurately portray the similarities and differences in views between typical IRBs and sex researchers. However, the empirical research in this area is extremely sparse. I provide references whenever possible, but, out of necessity, the current chapter is based on a blend of previous research and writings, personal experience, and informal accounts from colleagues, many of whom are members of the Society for the Scientific Study of Sexuality (SSSS). The relative dearth of citations in the current chapter is not meant to imply that research on these issues is unimportant or impossible (also see Farr & Seaver, 1975; Gergen, 1973; Stanley, Sieber, & Melton, 1987). In contrast, I hope to emphasize how future research might address the issues outlined, and it is my contention that it is a lack of empirical study that frequently has resulted in antagonism between sexuality researchers and IRBs (Mosher, 1988). I also highlight another neglected view—that of the research participant (Abramson, 1977; Milgram, 1977). I conclude by presenting some results from a pilot study I conducted on college student participants' reactions to sexuality research and by discussing some possible directions for future study.

IRB and Researcher Perspectives

In this culture, human sexuality is often considered a taboo topic. It should not be surprising that people, including one's academic colleagues, are prone to make a variety of attributions regarding professionals who could be labeled "sex researchers" (Brannigan, Allgeier, & Allgeier, 1997; Mosher, 1988). Unfortunately, peoples' notions of a sex researcher may entail negative attributions resulting in labels such as "voyeur" or "pervert." Against a backdrop of social taboo and possible suspicion regarding a sex researcher's motives, human beings serving as IRB members must make decisions regarding the ethical acceptability of proposed research. Accordingly, it should not be surprising that, compared to other research topics, IRBs frequently consider sexuality research to be a sensitive research area fraught with relatively more ethical concerns (Smith, Kaster-Bundgaard, & Council, 1996). In my experience, the primary IRB concerns with sexuality research involve issues of informed consent and potential harm to participants (also see Mosher, 1988).

Informed Consent

Most sexuality surveys conducted with college student samples, at least the ones from which the results are subsequently published in professional journals, appear to be anonymous. Accordingly, such anonymous paper-and-pencil surveys are exempt from the federal regulations regarding the protection of human subjects. Still, apparently because of the perceived sensitive nature of sexuality surveys, IRBs very often do not seem to treat such studies as truly exempt, and a written informed consent form is frequently required of researchers. In the context of a typical sexuality study with college student participants, informed consent primarily involves the issue of informing potential participants of the nature of the material they would encounter during the study (i.e., sexuality questions, attitudinal items, or sexual stimuli of some sort). I think that both researchers and IRB members would agree that providing adequate information to allow fully informed consent on the part of research participants is of utmost importance. Where disagreements frequently ensue is around the issue of the timing of such information and the level of disclosure provided. In other words, at what point will potential research participants be made aware that the study involves a sexual topic? To what degree will potential participants be made aware of the actual constructs measured in the study?

Both issues are important for the integrity of the results

generated by sexuality research. Many subject pools of which I am aware require researchers to post a brief description of the nature of the study along with the sign-up sheets. For a sexuality study the description may be as brief and generic as: "Participation in this study involves completing several questionnaires regarding your attitudes and experiences with intimate relationships" or may be relatively more revealing such as: "Participation in this study involves completing several questionnaires regarding your sexual attitudes and experiences." In either case, the researcher is likely to obtain a selective sample of college student participants. Others have convincingly shown that any indication that the study involves sexuality topics results in substantial self-selection on the part of students at the point of sign-up (Griffith & Walker, 1976; Jackson, Procidano, & Cohen, 1989). Those college students who sign up for the studies they believe to be sexual in nature are more likely to be male, extraverted, sensation-seeking, and sexually experienced.

One could criticize sexuality researchers for relying too heavily on college students and attempting to generalize to other adults. However, in many cases the college student samples on which sexuality research findings are based are themselves made up of a selective subgroup of college students represented by the subject pool. The issue of generalizability is probably much worse than it appears to those outside of the discipline. Also, infrequently is information about participant sign-up procedures provided in published reports to allow the reader to determine the extent to which self-selection might have been a problem.

If the issue only affected sex researchers, those not sympathetic to the endeavor might dismiss the issue as unimportant. However, the student self-selection that occurs with sexuality studies cuts both ways. If students are required (or desire) to participate in a certain number of studies, those types of students who shy away from sexuality studies will be overrepresented in studies not having to do with sexuality. In other words, we can expect that relatively introverted, conservative, sexually inexperienced students will comprise a larger proportion of the samples collected by researchers in other areas if a colleague is conducting sex research than if that colleague were not conducting sex research. It appears that this important sampling issue is infrequently recognized or appreciated.

In the ideal situation, at least from the researchers' perspective, student subject pool sign-up procedures would be such that student self-selection would be minimized. Regardless of the protocol, such self-selection will never be completely eliminated, especially in relatively small subject pools. That is, some students will disclose to peers the nature of the research study in which they participated, so the classmate may seek out or avoid certain studies based on word-of-mouth information. The problem would be minimized if students were not aware of the research topic at the point of sign-up, however. Without such awareness, how can researchers ensure informed consent and a lack of coercion to participate in particular studies?

One answer lies in the current protocol used for the subject pool in the department of psychological science at Ball State University. The posted sign-up sheets contain a code number assigned to the research project, the names of the researchers, the time and location of the study, whether the study involves a survey or an experiment, the amount of research credit being offered for participation, and any restrictions on potential participants (e.g., only males, only those with corrected 20/20 vision, etc.). Then, on arriving at the testing site, potential participants are given more detailed information about the nature of the project and what participation would entail. Those students who decide not to participate are given an opportunity to leave and seek out other ways to earn research participation credit, earning the minimum 30-minute unit of credit for having traveled to the testing site. In this way, each researcher can at least monitor the extent to which students appear to be self-selecting to participate in his or her particular project (although it is always possible, especially in smaller subject pools, that the code numbers associated with sexuality studies "leak out" to other students through word-of-mouth advertising from those students who have already participated).

What about coercion? It is possible that some students would feel too embarrassed to self-identify as someone uncomfortable with the research topic. It is also possible that some students might feel some (perhaps self-induced) pressure to participate after having signed up and arriving at the testing site. To counter these issues, I inform potential participants that they are free to decide not to participate now that they have learned the nature of the study, but, if they are uncomfortable leaving or participating, another option exists. Because the questionnaires are anonymous and will not be seen by the researcher until all participants have left the site, it is possible to "pretend" to participate, turn in a blank questionnaire when others turn in theirs, and then collect the credit.

By making potential participants aware of this option, I attempt to defuse the sampling problem without causing an additional problem involving perceived coercion. By giving those students who do not want to participate in a sexuality study the opportunity to receive research credit anyway, I hope to keep those individuals from being overrepresented in my colleagues' studies. As a side note, only about 1% of students in my studies to date have left the testing session on learning the nature of the study or have turned in a completely blank questionnaire. To the extent that sexuality researchers and IRBs disagree about the timing of informed consent when employing subject pools, compromise positions are available, such as those outlined previously, so that both student rights and research integrity are preserved. The second informed consent issue has to do with the level of disclosure to potential research participants regarding the constructs under study. Typically, researchers have no difficulty informing potential research participants that they will be asked to complete several widely used surveys designed to measure the respondent's sexual attitudes or will be asked to answer several questions regarding the respondent's sexual relationships. However, with regard to some constructs, divulging what is being measured would be detrimental to the integrity of the research project.

As an example, consider a project submitted for IRB approval by a graduate student whose thesis committee I chaired. Her proposed thesis project involved determining whether gender of the adult, gender of the child, or age of the child influenced perceptions that a sexual interaction involving an adult and child constituted child sexual abuse. Accordingly, each research participant would receive one version of a written narrative describing such a sexual interaction, and the age of the youth and the gender of the adult and youth would each be experimentally manipulated. The dependent variable was a rating by the research participant regarding the extent to which the respondent believed the depiction to be a case of child sexual abuse. Initially, the informed consent information to be provided to potential participants alerted them to the fact that participation involved reading a brief description of a sexual interaction and subsequently making judgments about it and the characters in the narrative. The IRB refused to approve the research unless potential participants were warned that they would be reading "a description of child sexual abuse."

It should be obvious that informing potential participants that they would be reading a depiction of child sexual abuse, and then subsequently asking them whether the depiction they read was a case of child sexual abuse, entails some serious methodological problems. Here was a case in which providing too much disclosure in the name of informed consent would have resulted in invalid research (and hence a waste of time for both the researcher and participants). The IRB's initial refusal to budge on this issue caused the student and I much distress (I will discuss the issue of emotional harm below) given that much labor had been invested in the proposed project and it had been approved by her thesis committee (which was made up of psychologists whom I believe to be of the highest ethical standards). In the end a compromise was reached, although it did not seem particularly satisfying to either "side." The student conducted the study, informing potential participants that they would encounter a description of "a sexual interaction involving an adult and a minor." The primary concern expressed by the

IRB involved potential harm to participants, an issue to which I now turn.

Harm to Participants

The federal guidelines regarding protection of human subjects define *minimal risk* such that the probability and magnitude of harm or discomfort anticipated in the research are not greater in and of themselves than those ordinarily encountered in daily life or during the performance of routine physical or psychological examinations or tests. In the current context, the issue is whether reading questionnaire items (or in the more extreme cases being exposed to some form of sexual stimuli) constitutes a greater probability and magnitude of harm or discomfort than the stresses of daily life or taking other psychological tests. Unfortunately, as objective criteria or data are sorely lacking, determining whether sexuality research constitutes more than minimal risk is a judgment call.

In this regard, it is interesting to note that, compared to more invasive types of research such as drug trials and hypnotic induction, IRBs appear to view sexuality surveys as posing relatively little risk of actual harm (Smith et al., 1996). However, among survey research topics, sexuality surveys seem to raise more concern than do surveys on less sensitive topics. In other words, I believe there is frequently a contrast phenomenon that occurs at many universities employing a subject pool. It is possible that at institutions at which the IRB routinely reviews proposals involving invasive procedures or drug trials, all questionnaire studies (even those involving sexuality topics) are viewed as relatively benign in contrast to those studies that present a risk of physical harm. However, at universities in which nearly all proposals reviewed by the IRB are psychological in nature, the contrast is more likely to occur between those surveys addressing more mundane topics (e.g., food preferences, leisure pursuits, academic experiences) and those that address relatively sensitive topics (e.g., sexuality, experience of traumatic events, history of antisocial behavior).

When the distinction is between relatively innocuous questionnaires versus those that deal with sexual topics, it is possible for IRB members to view the latter as somehow "riskier." Because reading questionnaire items cannot cause bodily harm (other than perhaps some eye strain under certain conditions), it appears that IRBs are concerned about emotional discomfort or psychological harm when the issue of potential harm to participants is raised (Mosher, 1988). Certainly that was the case with the graduate student whose interactions with the IRB I outlined earlier. The reason that the IRB required that the written informed consent form contain disclosure that participation involved reading a description of "child sexual abuse" was out of expressed concern for the psychological well-being of participants. The IRB expressed concern that some participants would have themselves experienced child sexual abuse, and that reading the brief description of a noninsertive sexual interaction between an adult and youth could cause substantial emotional discomfort or trauma to these individuals. I should note that the depiction had been used in at least two previously published studies with college students and the depiction did not include coercion or discussion of any type of response on the part of the youth. The IRB was aware of these points.

What was the probability that reading the depiction would result in psychological trauma for those students with a personal history of child sexual abuse? Unfortunately, despite the fact that this is an empirical question, no data exist (to my knowledge or that of my colleagues) regarding whether encountering written material such as that used in sexuality studies causes psychological discomfort. With a lack of empirical evidence, on what basis would an IRB member draw the conclusion that reading something in a sexuality questionnaire might result in harm? One potential answer has to do with scenario thinking. Cognitive psychologists have documented that humans are prone to scenario, or representative, thinking in which clusters of events or characteristics that can be imagined as belonging together are subsequently overestimated with regard to actual probability of occurrence (Dawes, 1988). In other words, if I can imagine a scenario in which a student (my imagination tells me probably female) who had been sexually abused as a child unwittingly reads the narrative describing the adult–youth sexual interaction and subsequently flashes on her own personal experience, resulting in anxiety and tears, I will tend to overestimate the likelihood of such a scenario actually occurring.

Given the relatively sensitive nature of sexual information in this culture, it is extremely difficult to anticipate how individuals will react to being asked certain questions about their sexual attitudes and experiences (even in an anonymous questionnaire). It is particularly difficult for any one individual to make such a determination, given that the individual has his or her own set of sexual attitudes and experiences and probably cannot help but be colored by them when making such a judgment. To make this judgment more problematic, in the context of college student subject pools the determination about effects of participation are being made by an IRB member who is clearly from a different generation from the potential research participants (who are typically 18 or 19 years of age), not to mention from a potentially different social background.

To offset the perceived potential harm in the form of emotional discomfort, IRBs frequently require sex researchers to include in a written informed consent form a statement similar to the following: "Participation in this research project may cause you some anxiety or emotional discomfort. If you experience uncomfortable emotions as a result of participating in this project, you are entitled to free counseling services at the university counseling center." Typically, participants are then given the telephone number and location of the counseling center. This warning and potential remedy are presented for the protection of participants, yet the effects of such a statement are unknown and apparently go unchallenged by researchers and IRB members alike.

It is conceivable that including such a statement actually causes some anxiety or sensitizes participants to the questionnaire material so that an emotional reaction of some sort is more likely. Medications contain an insert in which potential negative side-effects of taking the medication are listed.

These side-effects typically range from annoying symptoms to life-threatening events, and reading about their possible existence may cause substantial anxiety. However, the generation of such anxiety is apparently offset by the avoidance of serious medical complications that could result if the patient took the medication, had an adverse reaction, and was not aware of the potential for the side-effect. With psychological research, however, it is the anxiety or emotional discomfort itself that apparently is perceived by IRBs as the harm (Mosher, 1988). In this case, does it make sense to warn potential participants of possible anxiety if such a warning itself causes anxiety?

To my knowledge, no one has empirically investigated the emotional impact of such warning statements and attempts at remediation through directing the participant to counseling (nor has anyone investigated whether research participants ever seek out counseling as a result of participating in a study involving sexuality). However, Smith and Berard (1982) experimentally manipulated the description of a classic psychological study to examine how labeling potentially negative aspects of the study would affect college students' judgments about the research. The described study included both deception and possible psychological stress to participants. Each college student respondent read the same basic, accurate description of the study; however, in addition to the basic condition, one condition included labels inserted in the description (such as "deception" and "stress"), whereas another condition included an addendum instead (in which it was stated that "to relieve stress, subjects will be debriefed at the end of the experiment"). The college student respondents then answered several questions about the study, including whether it should be allowed by the university IRB, whether each would participate in the study, and whether any harm would be likely. The large majority of students indicated that the study should be allowed, that they would participate, and that no harm would result. However, compared to the basic condition, students in the label and addendum conditions were significantly less likely to indicate that the study should be approved by the IRB.

The implication of Smith and Berard's findings are important. It may be that, by alerting student participants to the potential for emotional discomfort, the study will be viewed more negatively than if the same study were conducted without highlighting the potential for emotional harm. It is interesting to note in this context that labeling the experiment as "deceptive" or involving "stress," or implying that such stress was likely through the need for debriefing, did not affect willingness to participate or degree of perceived harm associated with participation. In fact, the only effect of such labeling was with regard to judgments about the acceptability of the study to the IRB. It is possible that sex researchers, by trying to anticipate IRB members' concerns over perceived emotional "harm," actually make their proposed studies less acceptable to IRBs by explicitly labeling the possibility for anxiety or discomfort. Of course much more empirical study is needed to address the potential effects of warnings and references to the provision of counseling services on both participants' and IRB members' judgments of proposed sexuality studies.

The Participant Perspective

Determining the extent to which participating in a sexuality study will cause the college student participants some degree of emotional discomfort exceeding that encountered in daily living requires assessing the actual effects of such participation as perceived by the participants themselves. Despite the important implications of such research, it is nearly nonexistent. I was able to locate only one report on the perceptions of research participants in sexuality research.

Abramson (1977) conducted a study involving 40 men and 40 women from an introductory psychology subject pool. Participation involved completing an anonymous questionnaire regarding sexual experiences and sexual attitudes, reading an erotic story and rating one's subsequent sexual arousal, being secretly observed in a waiting room containing sexually explicit magazines, responding to double-entendre words, and being tested for retention of information presented on reproductive biology. Subsequent to participating in all phases of the study, participants were invited to attend a debriefing session in which a brief lecture was presented on correlational research, the measures used in the study were described, the distribution of participant responses to each measure were described, the procedures and deception were explained, and references for all pertinent previous studies were provided. Certainly, both the study and the debriefing procedure were extraordinary. Important for the current context, Abramson also had participants complete an anonymous questionnaire after the debriefing regarding their perceptions of having participated in the project.

Based on the results, Abramson (1977) concluded that "participation was viewed as an enjoyable learning experience which produced no negative aftereffects. In fact, the overwhelming agreement among subjects indicates that the measures employed to safeguard ethical requirements were sufficient to induce a very positive regard for the experimental procedures. It is also interesting to note that not a single subject felt that any part of this experiment was a serious invasion of privacy" (p. 189). The large majority of participants in Abramson's study judged their participation to be an important learning experience and a significant contribution to sexual science. These results are encouraging, but most sex researchers do not provide the extensive debriefing–educational session Abramson did. Also, as mentioned earlier, one cannot generalize to the student subject pool at large, because the participants in Abramson's (1977) study initially signed up to participate in a study advertised as having to do with sexual attitudes and behavior (see p. 186).

The participants in Abramson's study deemed their research experience to be a positive one. However, they had likely self-selected and were probably more comfortable with sexual topics than were their subject pool peers who did not sign up for the study. Also, we do not know whether perceived comfort or discomfort during participation is related to likelihood of participating in a similar study in the future. If discomfort and likelihood of future participation are unrelated, perhaps participants are not placing much importance on emotional discomfort as the criterion for determining whether to participate in a particular study (as would be implied by IRB concerns over informed consent about potential discomfort). To address some of these issues in at least a rudimentary way, I recently conducted the following assessment of college student participants' perceptions.

The primary focus of the survey administered to 310 men and 399 women recruited from the psychological science subject pool at Ball State University was experiences of extradyadic involvement during courtship. In other words, each respondent was asked extensively about instances in which he or she was involved in a serious dating relationship with one person yet concurrently engaged in a variety of dating and sexual experiences with someone else. As potential correlates of such extradyadic experience, several other variables were measured, including demographic information, religiosity, self-monitoring, relationship style, body satisfaction and self-rated physical attractiveness, sexual attitudes, sexual esteem, sexual sensation seeking, and recent and lifetime sexual experience (sexual intercourse, oral sex, casual sex). In many respects the anonymous 10-page survey created for this study was typical of those used in sexuality research with college student subject pools. At the end of the survey respondents were asked to self-rate the "comfort level while participating in this study" using a 5-point scale (1 = *very uncomfortable*, 2 = *uncomfortable*, 3 = *not really affected*, 4 = *comfortable*, 5 = *very comfortable*). Respondents were also asked, in a yes or no format, "Would you participate in another sexuality study involving an anonymous questionnaire if given the opportunity to do so in the future?"

Given my earlier emphasis on possible self-selection at the point of sign-up, as well as potential effects of implying that participation may cause anxiety, it is important to note that participants in the current study were unaware of the sexual nature of the study at the point of initial sign-up, and they were provided with verbal informed consent in which no mention was made of potential anxiety or provision of counseling services to combat any ill effects from participation.

The two research assistants who conducted the study reported that no one left the numerous testing sessions on learning of the nature of the questionnaire. I hope, then, that the current sample fairly represents the students involved in the subject pool during that particular semester. Also, it is important to note that even though extradyadic involvement during courtship is considered a socially undesirable behavior (Lieberman, 1988; Sheppard, Nelson, & Andreoli-Mathie, 1995), relatively large numbers of respondents in the current study reported such experience. So one might expect relatively high levels of discomfort responding to questions about a taboo topic, especially when one admits to socially undesirable behavior.

Taking a rating of 1 or 2 as indicative of some discomfort, a rating of 3 as neutral, and a rating of 4 or 5 as indicative of a positive response, 19.7% of the men and 24.3% of the women indicated some level of discomfort during the study. A positive response was most common (54.8% of men and 45.8% of women). Still, there was a sizeable minority of respondents (about one in five) who reported some discomfort during participation. One might imagine that if these respondents experienced discomfort, they would be hesitant to participate in a similar study in the future. However, 97.4% of the men and 94.7% of the women indicated that they would indeed complete an anonymous questionnaire regarding sexuality if given the opportunity in the future.

As one might expect, a smaller proportion (89.9%) of the respondents who were relatively uncomfortable would volunteer for a similar study in the future compared to respondents whose emotional reaction was neutral or positive (97.6%; χ^2 [1, $N = 709$] = 18.88, $p < .0001$). However, rates of volunteering for a future study were actually slightly *higher* for respondents who reported having experienced extradyadic dating (97.8%) compared to those who denied such experience (94.7%; χ^2 [1, $N = 708$] = 3.90, $p < .05$). The rates of volunteering among those respondents who reported extradyadic sexual intercourse and those who denied such activity did not differ (95.5% versus 96.1%, respectively; χ^2 [1, $N = 709$] = .17, $p < .69$). Also, increasing levels of comfort while participating in the study were related to relatively greater numbers of lifetime sex partners, more liberal sexual attitudes, and greater sexual esteem and sexual sensation seeking. So, had participants self-selected at the point of initial sign-up, presumably those respondents who indicated the most discomfort would have avoided the study, resulting in a less representative sample.

Conclusion

Research on sexuality is frequently seen as ethically riskier than research involving similar methodology but focusing on a less sensitive topic. When college student subject pools are involved, IRBs appear to be most commonly concerned about informed consent and potential emotional harm to participants. Despite the fact that the federal guidelines for the protection of human subjects declares anonymous questionnaires as exempt from the policy, sexuality studies based on such questionnaires are frequently treated as somehow riskier, and in need of greater IRB control, than the federal guidelines necessarily dictate. Conflicts are liable to ensue between researchers and IRBs with regard to issues of potential harm and steps needed to protect participants from such perceived harm (Mosher, 1988). Compromise positions are frequently reached, yet greater empirical study on several issues raised in this chapter would help resolve some of the ongoing debate (Stanley et al., 1987).

What are the effects of informed consent forms, warnings about potential emotional discomfort, and information about possible counseling resources on college student participants in sexuality studies? To what degree does the experience of emotional discomfort during sexuality studies differ from that experienced during more mundane studies (Farr & Seaver, 1975), or from daily stresses (particularly for college students who frequently appear to be more stressed out about exams and educational requirements than about anonymous questionnaires)? How do the individual characteristics of college students and IRB members influence respective judgments about the appropriateness and potential harm of sexuality studies? These are just a few of the important empirical questions that need to be addressed in future research. Because IRBs cannot be expected to conduct these studies, it is incumbent on those engaged in sexuality research to begin evaluating the perceptions others have of their research and the effects their research has on participants.

In closing, I would like to offer a few suggestions for those individuals involved in administration of subject pools, those serving on IRBs, and those conducting studies related to human sexuality. In overseeing a subject pool it is easy to "play it safe" and require complete disclosure of the nature and details of studies at the point of sign-up. However, I urge you to consider the biases introduced when one does so. One of the primary benefits of a student subject pool is the educational opportunities it affords students. Certainly, explaining to students the reasons for the limited information at sign-up should make sense to them and will illustrate important points about sampling and bias. I perceive students as generally caring about whether their research participation makes a difference and contributes to a larger scientific enterprise. If students knew that the validity of the projects in which they were participating was being compromised by certain sign-up procedures, some students may be angered (or at least disappointed).

I urge individuals serving on IRBs to resist the human tendency to engage in scenario thinking or to base one's judgments on a personal frame of reference. Both sources of decision making are liable to be at odds with the world as it exists for others. As Mosher (1988) noted, "Appointment to [an IRB] is not, in itself, a sufficient preparation for making informed and fair ethical judgments" (p. 382). Indeed, we all should continually consult the federal guidelines for protection of human subjects. Also, in making judgments about whether a proposed study is exempt from such federal guidelines, one needs to remember that such a judgment is based on the methodology (e.g., anonymous questionnaire) rather than the topic of the study (Mosher, 1988). Last, to remain fair to both participants as well as researchers, criticisms and required modifications of proposed projects should be based on citations to particular portions of the federal guidelines or ethics code being used.

To researchers conducting sexuality studies with subject pools, I urge consideration of the sampling biases I discussed earlier. If constrained by current policies, researchers should at least detail in their research reports the method of recruiting participants (e.g., sign-up sheet procedures). I also urge researchers to take up the task of applying their empirical skills to understanding the experience of research participants (Stanley et al., 1987). Many of the issues raised in the current chapter would not be debatable had previous researchers evaluated the effects of conducting research on participants and the attributions and judgments participants make regarding the process (e.g., Wilson & Donnerstein, 1976). Armed with such data, we could alter our methodology as needed for more ethically sound research and assist IRBs in making more informed decisions regarding research proposals. Ideally, the relationship between researchers and IRBs would be a collaborative one in which the interests of participant protection and research integrity would be paramount for both.

References

Abramson, P. R. (1977). Ethical requirements for research on human sexual behavior: From the perspective of participating subjects. *Journal of Social Issues, 33*, 184–192.

Brannigan, G. G., Allgeier, A. R., & Allgeier, E. R. (1997). *The sex scientists.* New York: Addison-Wesley.

Dawes, R. M. (1988). *Rational choice in an uncertain world.* New York: Harcourt Brace Jovanovich.

Farr, J. L., & Seaver, W. B. (1975). Stress and discomfort in psychological research: Subject perceptions of experimental procedures. *American Psychologist, 30*, 770–773.

Gergen, K. J. (1973). The codification of research ethics: Views of a doubting Thomas. *American Psychologist, 28*, 907–912.

Griffith, M., & Walker, C. E. (1976). Characteristics associated with expressed willingness to participate in psychological research. *Journal of Social Psychology, 100,* 157–158.

Jackson, J. M., Procidano, M. E., & Cohen, C. J. (1989). Subject pool sign-up procedures: A threat to external validity. *Social Behavior and Personality, 17,* 29–43.

Lieberman, B. (1988). Extrapremarital intercourse: Attitudes toward a neglected sexual behavior. *The Journal of Sex Research, 24,* 291–299.

Milgram, S. (1977). Subject reaction: The neglected factor in the ethics of experimentation. *Hastings Center Report, 7,* 19–23.

Mosher, D. L. (1988). Balancing the rights of subjects, scientists, and society: 10 principles for human subject committees. *The Journal of Sex Research, 24,* 378–385.

Sheppard, V. J., Nelson, E. S., & Andreoli-Mathie, V. (1995). Dating relationships and infidelity: Attitudes and behaviors. *Journal of Sex & Marital Therapy, 21,* 202–212.

Smith, C. P., & Berard, S. P. (1982). Why are human subjects less concerned about ethically problematic research than human subjects committees? *Journal of Applied Social Psychology, 12,* 209–221.

Smith, E. J. H., Kaster-Bundgaard, J., & Council, J. R. (1996, May). *Getting along with your IRB: A practical guide for researchers.* Poster presented at the annual meeting of the Midwestern Psychological Association, Chicago.

Stanley, B., Sieber, J. E., & Melton, G. B. (1987). Empirical studies of ethical issues in research: A research agenda. *American Psychologist, 42,* 735–741.

Wilson, D. W., & Donnerstein, E. (1976). Legal and ethical aspects of nonreactive social psychological research: An excursion into the public mind. *American Psychologist, 31,* 765–773.

Index

harm to participants, 208–212
IRBs and, 8, 202–212
participant perspectives, 212–216
reliance on self-report, 201
researcher perspectives, 202–212
Shoben, Edward, 131*n*, 151–152
Social desirability, 111–112
Society for the Scientific Study of Sexuality (SSSS), 202
Structuralism, 3
Subject pool application packets, 89–90
Subject pools. *See* Department subject pools
Subjects' rights initiatives, 159–160

SUNY Brockport, 168, 173

Teaching, 172–173
Telephone reminder, 119–123
Tuskegee syphilis experiments, 160

ULRICH's serial directory, 69
University of Illinois (UI) at Urbana-Champaign, 133
University of Pittsburgh, 88

Voluntary participation, 48, 51–52, 70

Way finding, 115, 118, 124
Wiederman, Michael W., 201
Wiretapping, 159–160

About the Editors

Garvin Chastain received his PhD in human experimental psychology from the University of Texas at Austin in 1976. He joined the faculty of Boise State University in 1978, where he was Coordinator of General Psychology for 10 years, and currently is Professor of Psychology. He has received distinguished teaching and distinguished faculty awards as well as honors in teaching and special faculty recognition awards from Boise State University. He is a Fellow of the Western Psychological Association.

He was instrumental in establishing a human subject pool at Boise State University, and has headed the Psychology Department's Human Subject Pool Committee since 1993. He has published more than 60 articles in refereed professional journals. His research interest is visual cognition, and includes topics related to pattern recognition and visual spatial attention. He is executive editor of *The Journal of General Psychology*, an associate editor of *The Journal of Psychology*, and serves on the editorial advisory board of *Genetic, Social, and General Psychology Monographs*.

R. Eric Landrum is Associate Professor and Chair of the Department of Psychology at Boise State University in Boise, Idaho. He received his PhD from Southern Illinois University—Carbondale. His research interests center around educational issues and how college students can maximize their university experience. Examples of specific areas of research interest include understanding student study time, grade inflation, how students use textbooks, and student evaluations of teaching effectiveness. In addition, he has an interest in the use of the World Wide Web, especially in the area of survey design and data collection, and a general research interest in the role of surveys in changing and affecting behavior (e.g., venting), as well as an interest in creating a general psychology course for Internet / CD-ROM users. He has numerous conference presentations and publications to his credit, and serves as a consulting editor for *Teaching of Psychology* and the *Journal of General Psychology*, and as an ad hoc reviewer for the *Journal of Marriage and the Family* and the *Psi Chi Journal of Undergraduate Research*. He is a member of the American Psychological Association, Midwestern Psychological Association, Phi Kappa Phi, Sigma Xi, Idaho Academy of Sciences, American Society for Training and Development, and he is the national president-elect of the Council of Teachers of Undergraduate Psychology (CTUP).